Perimenopause Mindset

A Psychologist's Guide to Rewiring Habits, Stopping Emotional Eating, and Lasting Mental Health

Priscilla Leitner

Published by Eloria Press Orlando, Florida

First edition, 2026

ISBN 979-8-9963491-0-4

Editorial direction: Eloria Press
Interior design: Eloria Press
Cover design: Eloria Press

This book is intended for educational purposes only and does not replace medical, psychological, or professional healthcare advice, diagnosis, or treatment. Readers should consult qualified healthcare professionals regarding individual health concerns.

Instagram: @eloriapress

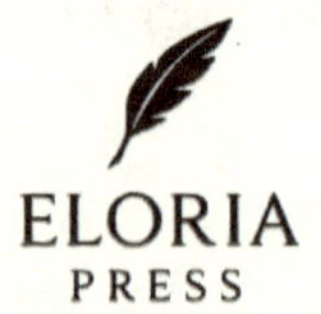

Table of Contents

Introduction

It often begins as a whisper, not a shout. One day, you're powering through your calendar, managing both your work deadlines and your family's schedules with practiced efficiency. Then, out of nowhere, things start to feel different. You wake up at 3:00 a.m., mind racing over every detail from the day before. That afternoon, you snap at a colleague over something you wouldn't normally notice. Later, you find yourself staring into the fridge, wondering if another handful of snacks will fix an emptiness you can't quite name. Some days, it all feels manageable. Other days, the ground beneath your routines feels like it's shifting out of control.

If you've found yourself puzzling over these changes, you're far from alone.

For millions of women in their late 30s through early 50s, perimenopause sets in quietly, yet changes everything. Even if you're high-achieving and health-conscious, you might find yourself caught off guard. You might laugh nervously about "brain fog" or sudden mood swings, but do you really understand how deeply this transition can affect your focus, emotions, and sense of control?

Maybe you've told yourself you're "just stressed" or that the changes in sleep, energy, appetite, and focus will pass. Perhaps you've stayed up late Googling advice that only left you more confused. You might've even tried harder to eat cleaner, exercise more, or think positively, hoping to hold things together. If any of this sounds like your journey, know that you're not imagining things, and you're certainly not failing. Your body and mind are sending real signals that deserve understanding.

It's time to address the worries many women share but rarely say out loud: *Am I still myself if I don't feel like myself? Will anyone take me seriously if I admit I'm struggling? Does this mean I'm getting old, or losing value?* The truth is that perimenopause isn't a disorder or a decline. It's a natural, meaningful transition in your biology and identity. The unpredictability of symptoms and the feeling like you're losing control are part of a shared human experience. When you understand what's happening, you can respond with compassion and strength.

This book is an invitation to make sense of these changes, with science and compassion as your guides. You won't find quick fixes, scare tactics, or patronizing advice. Instead, you'll learn to see perimenopause as a window for renewal. When you use this time intentionally, you can reduce symptom intensity later in menopause and build steadier foundations for physical, emotional, behavioral, and relational well-being.

Through the framework of the six pillars of the Perimenopause Mindset, you'll learn how to stabilize your daily rhythms, strengthen self-regulation, and prepare your body and mind for a lighter transition into menopause. You'll find gentle approaches for emotional balance, tools that restore resilience rather than deplete it, and communication tips for more productive healthcare conversations. More importantly, you'll gain freedom from shame, guilt, and the myth that perfection is the answer. Together, we'll replace self-criticism with curiosity and self-awareness, shifting from "fixing" to thriving.

I want you to know who's walking alongside you on this journey. My name is Dr. Priscilla Leitner. I'm a clinical psychologist in Brazil, specializing in eating behavior, lifestyle, and mental health. For the past two decades, I've trained clinicians, mentored clients, and built a research institute advancing the science of eating behavior, eating disorders, and lifestyle. For years, I saw intelligent, capable women struggling during midlife, feeling disoriented by changes no one had prepared them for. Experiencing these changes in my own body encouraged me to write this book to help you navigate those uncertain feelings.

My work blends science with empathy. I believe that real transformation happens when research meets self-compassion. *Perimenopause Mindset* continues on that mission, helping you understand what's happening, take back your agency, and design a more intentional life at midlife and beyond.

To guide you clearly but gently, this book starts by clearing away myths, then explores how shifting hormones affect your body, brain, and mood. You'll learn about the my six core pillars for a lifestyle that's emotionally sustainable: eating, movement, stress, sleep, emotional regulation, and imbalances, and how to apply them to restore balance today while protecting your well-being for the years ahead. Later, you'll focus on medical care, habit rewiring, and daily rhythms that promote long-term clarity and calm. Every section offers actionable insights that fit within busy schedules, so you never have to choose between taking care of others and caring for yourself.

This book won't ask you to deny your discomfort or pretend that everything is fine. Perimenopause is complex. Your biology, your thoughts, your beliefs, and your surroundings are all connected. The approaches here blend medical knowledge, psychological perspective, and real-life wisdom, helping you restore that connection so that you can feel grounded, capable, and in control again. There's no single "right" path forward, but many ways to thrive. You get to choose which ones feel right for you.

Think of this as your reset button: a structured yet compassionate process that stabilizes your rhythms, strengthens resilience, and prepares you for a smoother, more empowered transition into menopause. Each chapter is designed with both information and compassion in mind. You'll find ideas that challenge outdated beliefs and small experiments that create genuine progress. Turning this page is your first act of self-leadership and a reminder that your well-being matters. You already have what it takes to meet this season of life with courage and curiosity.

I invite you to read at your own pace. Pause, reflect, jot down what resonates, and experiment gently. Don't worry about getting it perfect. Some days you'll take bold steps, while other days, you may feel uncertain. That's okay. Self-compassion will be your most reliable tool, helping you move forward even when things feel hard.

Throughout this book, you can expect honesty without alarmism, encouragement without fluff, and strategies grounded in research. You'll see yourself reflected in these pages as someone capable of great adaptability, courage, and growth. While there may be difficult moments, there's also an immense opportunity and an open door to recalibrate your health, rediscover your strengths, and redefine what thriving means for you.

Welcome to *Perimenopause Mindset,* a new conversation about midlife, grounded in science, guided by empathy, and written with you in mind.

Part I:

Wake Up and Grounding

(Weeks 1 to 2)

Chapter 1:

Understanding Perimenopause—Clear Signs, Myths, and Why This Moment Matters

Have you noticed your energy changing in ways that you can't quite explain? Do your moods feel different from what you're used to, even when life around you has stayed the same? Have your sleep patterns shifted or become harder to predict? Do your periods seem less familiar than they once were? Many women begin sensing these shifts years before they learn that they are part of a normal transition called perimenopause.

Let's take a close look at perimenopause, the phase of life leading to menopause that many women experience but few fully understand. We'll explore how to recognize the clear signs and symptoms, both physical and emotional, so you can better tune in to what your body is telling you. Along the way, we'll unpack some of the myths and misunderstandings surrounding this time, helping dissolve the shame that many women carry in silence. We'll also look at why perimenopause can be a reset point, a time to strengthen daily rhythms, and build habits that support long-term well-being.

Understanding Perimenopause as a Reset Window

Perimenopause is the gradual transition that leads up to menopause. It typically begins in your late 30s or early 40s, though some women experience it earlier or later. It can affect you for anything between four and eight years, or even more, before you go into full menopause. During this stage, the ovaries start producing estrogen and progesterone in irregular patterns. These fluctuations affect many systems in the body, including temperature regulation, sleep, mood, cognition, metabolism, and emotional resilience.

Although the symptoms can feel unpredictable, this phase is a natural biological process, and within it lies a unique opportunity for you. When you make the most of this time, you can change your future and reduce the severity of menopause.

That is why I firmly believe that perimenopause is more than a hormonal shift. It's your built-in window for renewal. During this time, your body becomes especially responsive to supportive habits and stabilizing rhythms.

This reset isn't a quick fix. It is a structured and compassionate process that strengthens your daily routines, enhances emotional and metabolic regulation, and prepares your system for a smoother, lighter transition into menopause. Understanding what is happening in your body helps replace fear with clarity. When you approach this season with intention rather than urgency, you reclaim agency in a stage of life that often leaves women feeling overwhelmed, confused, or dismissed.

This reset window is about creating stability where hormones create instability, and about building practices that support you long after the transition is complete. It's a chance to realign your rhythms, nourish yourself differently, and enter the next chapter of your life with greater steadiness and self-leadership.

Recognizing Early Physical Changes

Perimenopause often begins with subtle shifts in the body that can feel confusing if you aren't expecting them. These changes reflect the natural decline and fluctuation of estrogen and progesterone, which influence multiple systems, including reproductive, metabolic, and thermoregulatory functions (Santoro et al., 2015). Early recognition gives you the chance to respond gently and intentionally, rather than reacting with worry. Some of the most common physical symptoms include (*Perimenopause*, 2025):

Menstrual Changes

- Periods may become irregular, arriving earlier or later than usual.
- Bleeding may fluctuate in volume, sometimes heavier and other times lighter than expected.
- Cycle length can shorten for several months, then lengthen again unpredictably.
- Skipping cycles intermittently is common and usually reflects hormonal adjustments rather than underlying illness.

Hot Flashes and Night Sweats

- Sudden warmth, often starting in the chest, neck, or face, may cause flushing or sweating.
- Night sweats can disrupt sleep and leave you feeling fatigued during the day.
- Severity varies: some women experience mild warmth, and others need changes in clothing or bedding.

Sleep Disruptions

- Falling asleep or staying asleep may become more difficult.

- Waking in the early morning hours and struggling to return to sleep is common.
- These sleep changes are closely linked to fluctuating hormone levels, which affect the body's circadian rhythms and thermoregulation.

Skin, Hair, and Body Changes

- Skin may feel drier, more sensitive, or develop a papery texture.
- Hair can thin, lose shine, or become more brittle.
- Some women notice changes in body temperature perception, such as feeling colder or warmer than usual.

Becoming more aware of these physical signals allows you to track patterns, communicate clearly with healthcare providers, and implement lifestyle practices that will help you use this stage of your life as a reset.

Understanding Emotional and Cognitive Shifts

Perimenopause doesn't just affect you physically, but emotionally and mentally as well. This stage of life can bring noticeable changes in your mood, emotional regulation, and cognitive function (Digitale, 2024). These shifts are due to the ways in which fluctuating estrogen and progesterone influence neurotransmitters that regulate your mood, focus, and memory. Here are common symptoms to look out for (Dutchen, 2021):

Mood and Emotional Regulation

- Irritability can increase, sometimes triggered by minor stressors that previously felt manageable.

- Anxiety may become more prominent, making everyday responsibilities feel more overwhelming.
- Rapid mood swings can occur, with emotions changing from hopeful and happy to sad or frustrated in a short period.
- Understanding that hormones affect emotions allows you to respond with self-compassion rather than self-criticism.

Cognitive Changes

- "Brain fog" may appear, making it harder to recall names, keep track of keys, or remember details in meetings.
- Processing information can feel slower, and multitasking may become more challenging.
- These cognitive shifts are temporary and often improve with strategies that support executive function, such as keeping lists, practicing mindfulness, and prioritizing sleep.

Behavioral Responses

- Emotional eating can increase as a way to cope with stress or low mood.
- Impulsive reactions may occur more frequently in high-pressure situations.
- Pausing to recognize these patterns helps reduce shame and allows for gentle habit adjustments, such as mindful snacking or short breaks for movement or breathing exercises.

Awareness of these emotional and cognitive patterns creates space for you to implement strategies that enhance your stability, reduce stress, and boost your confidence in work, relationships, and daily life.

Less Common but Important Symptoms

While you may notice changes in cycles, mood, and sleep, perimenopause can also bring subtler shifts that are easily overlooked. Recognizing these early helps you respond proactively rather than feeling uncertain or alarmed. Some of the symptoms you may experience can be:

Libido and Sexual Health

- Sexual desire may fluctuate, sometimes declining without an obvious external reason.
- Vaginal dryness or discomfort during intimacy can emerge as estrogen levels change.

Joint, Muscle, and Bone Changes

- Some women notice joint aches or stiffness, especially in the mornings or after light activity.
- Maintaining movement and strength exercises now can protect bone and muscle health in the years ahead.

Digestive and Metabolic Changes

- Digestion may become less predictable, with bloating or discomfort after foods previously tolerated well.
- Metabolism may shift gradually, sometimes contributing to weight changes even without dietary or activity changes.

Temperature Regulation and Sensory Shifts

- Hands and feet may feel colder or warmer than usual, often with no clear reason.

- Some women experience heightened sensitivity to smells, tastes, or textures.

Tracking these subtler changes gives you the insight to implement adjustments gradually, reinforcing a sense of control.

How Myths Shape Your Experience

You've probably heard some stories about perimenopause that make it sound scary or impossible to manage. Maybe friends, ads, or TV shows make it seem like everything in your life, including your energy, your mood, and your body, will suddenly go downhill. The truth is, these stories often exaggerate challenges and feed unnecessary shame. Recognizing myth versus reality lets you focus on practical steps and celebrate your small wins.

Common Myths

- Some people say perimenopause is just a slow slide into decline, where you lose energy, focus, or even attractiveness. The reality is that these experiences vary widely, and you may feel fine or even empowered during this phase.

- You might hear that any weight gain or body changes are unavoidable and your fault. While hormones do influence metabolism, your lifestyle, stress, and genetics all play a role, small, consistent habits make meaningful differences over time.

- Another myth is that mood swings or irritability mean you've lost control. Often, these shifts are simply your brain and hormones adjusting. Noticing your emotions without judgment is part of progress.

Impact of Myths

- Believing these myths can make you second-guess yourself or feel guilty about normal changes.

- You might delay asking for help, trying new habits, or talking to your doctor because you feel you "should" be handling everything perfectly.
- Internalizing these stories can make perimenopause feel isolating, like you're the only one struggling, when in reality, millions of women experience similar shifts during this phase of their lives.

Reframing the Narrative

Perimenopause isn't a problem to hide, but rather a natural life phase that can be challenging at times, but comes with many opportunities to make lasting changes to your life. When you recognize which stories are myths, you can respond with curiosity instead of judgment.

Understanding the reality of perimenopause allows you to make decisions based on what actually works for your body, rather than what culture tells you should happen.

Why Shame Persists

Even when you know the facts, it's common to feel a little embarrassed about what's happening during perimenopause, or even like you need to keep your experience a secret. That shame often comes from the stories society tells about this phase of life, and not enough women speak up about what they're really going through.

Many women feel like they should be handling it all perfectly. Struggling with weight changes, mood swings, or cravings for comfort food can easily trigger guilt or self-criticism. You might catch yourself thinking, "I shouldn't be this tired," or "I shouldn't feel this way." These thoughts make it tempting to hide your experiences, avoid talking to friends, or even put off appointments with your doctor.

Shame also sticks because of societal silence. Health classes, mainstream media, and public conversations rarely cover perimenopause in depth. Many women enter this phase without even knowing what to expect. When you don't see your experience reflected anywhere, it's easy to believe you're "doing it wrong."

The good news is that understanding the biology behind these shifts can melt that shame away. Mood swings, forgetfulness, night sweats, or sudden cravings are the natural result of changing hormone levels. When you can name what's happening, it's easier to replace judgment with compassion. Instead of thinking, "Something is wrong with me," you can shift to, "My body is adapting, and these feelings are temporary."

When you have accurate information and a clear understanding of what's happening in your body, you can let go of that shame. That clarity gives you the freedom to ask for help, try new strategies, and build habits that actually support your health and well-being. Recognizing that perimenopause is a normal, shared experience can turn isolation into connection and uncertainty into proactive care. It can turn perimenopause into the reset it can be.

Reframing Perimenopause as a Turning Point

Perimenopause is more than just uncomfortable symptoms and challenges. It's an invitation to pause, reflect, and take charge of your health in a new way. Instead of seeing it as a decline, think of it as a chance to reset your habits, routines, and priorities.

Your body is sending signals for a reason. Changes in sleep, energy, or mood are nudges to pay attention. When you respond with intention, you can turn these shifts into opportunities. Maybe you need more rest, a different approach to movement, or a new way to manage stress. Small adjustments now can have a big impact, helping you feel more grounded today and easing the transition into menopause later.

This phase is also a chance to experiment with habits that support long-term well-being. Eating more mindfully, moving in ways that energize rather than exhaust you, or practicing brief moments of mindfulness each day can all become anchors. Each choice is a step toward greater resilience, clarity, and self-trust.

By reframing perimenopause as a turning point, you stop fighting your body and start working with it. You reclaim a sense of agency and transform uncertainty into curiosity. What feels like disruption can become a doorway to a more intentional, empowered midlife.

Developing a Growth Mindset

How you think about perimenopause shapes your experience more than you might realize. Approaching this phase with a growth mindset and believing that challenges are opportunities to learn and adapt can make a big difference in your emotional and physical well-being.

Instead of seeing mood swings, sleep disruption, or cravings as obstacles or evidence that something is "wrong," a growth mindset frames them as signals. They are clues that your body and brain are adjusting, and that small, intentional changes can create meaningful improvement. For example, noticing that your energy dips in the afternoon might inspire a new snack, a brief walk, or a mindful pause that actually boosts focus and mood.

Research shows that people who adopt a growth mindset experience less stress, higher resilience, and better problem-solving when facing change. In the context of perimenopause, this perspective encourages curiosity rather than judgment, experimentation instead of self-blame, and gradual progress in place of perfectionism.

Here are a few tips for cultivating a growth mindset during perimenopause:

- **Reframe challenges as experiments:** Instead of saying, "I can't handle this," try, "This is a chance to see what works for me."

- **Track small wins:** Keep a journal of small improvements in sleep, energy, mood, or cravings to reinforce progress over time.

- **Practice self-compassion:** Talk to yourself as you would to a friend. Mistakes and setbacks are normal, not failures.

- **Ask reflective questions:** "What can I learn from this day?" or "What adjustment might make this easier next time?" encourages insight rather than frustration.

- **Celebrate adaptability:** Recognize when you try a new strategy or make a positive change, even if results aren't immediate.

Embracing growth doesn't remove your challenges, but it gives you the tools to face them with adaptability and optimism. When you combine knowledge of your body with a mindset that values learning and flexibility, perimenopause becomes a season of insight, empowerment, and personal growth.

Tools to Begin Your Reset

Perimenopause is a time of awareness, reflection, and intentional action. These tools are designed to help you tune into your body, track patterns, and start shifting your mindset so you can navigate this phase with clarity and confidence.

Symptom Checklist

Tracking your perimenopause symptoms helps you see patterns, understand your body, and communicate more effectively with your healthcare provider. Use this checklist daily or weekly, noting the intensity or frequency of each symptom. You can rate them on a simple scale of 0 = none, 1 = mild, 2 = moderate, 3 = severe.

Physical symptoms:

▢ menstrual cycle changes (earlier, later, heavier, lighter, skipped cycles) ______

▢ hot flashes or sudden warmth _______

▢ night sweats or disrupted sleep _______

▢ changes in skin, hair, or nails _______

▢ joint aches or stiffness _______

▢ digestive changes, bloating, or discomfort _______

▢ changes in libido _______

Emotional symptoms:

▢ mood swings _______

▢ irritability or anger _______

▢ anxiety or restlessness _______

▢ overwhelm or low mood _______

▢ cravings or emotional eating _______

Cognitive symptoms:

▢ brain fog or forgetfulness _______

▢ trouble focusing or following conversations _______

▢ slower processing of information _______

Other observations:

▢ energy levels throughout the day _______

▢ elevated stress _______

▢ relationship or communication challenges _______

▢ self-care habits (exercise, nutrition, or relaxation) _______

Tips for using the checklist:

- Track symptoms for at least two weeks to notice patterns.
- Write notes beside each symptom to add context, such as triggers or circumstances.
- Bring your completed checklist to appointments with healthcare providers to have more productive conversations.
- Use it as a starting point for reflection prompts, journaling, or mindful check-ins.

Reflection Prompts

After tracking your symptoms for a few days or weeks, take a moment to pause and reflect. These prompts are designed to help you explore your experience, notice patterns, and start thinking about intentional changes. Write your answers in a journal or notebook.

Understanding Your Body

What physical symptoms have been most noticeable or surprising to me?

____

____

____

____

____

When do these symptoms tend to appear, and are there patterns related to time of day, stress, or activity?

How do my energy levels fluctuate throughout the day?

Emotional Awareness

Which emotions feel strongest right now, and how do they show up in my daily life?

Are there situations that consistently trigger irritability, anxiety, or sadness?

How do I currently respond to these feelings, and how would I like to react differently?

Cognitive Patterns

Which mental challenges feel most present, such as brain fog, forgetfulness, or difficulty focusing?

Are there specific strategies I have used that help improve focus or recall?

How can I integrate these strategies more consistently?

____

____

____

____

Mindset and Self-Compassion

What stories or beliefs about perimenopause have I noticed in my thinking?

____

____

____

____

How can I reframe challenges as opportunities for growth rather than evidence of loss?

____

____

____

____

What small acts of self-compassion can I practice today to honor my body and mind?

____

____

Looking Ahead

Which habits or routines feel supportive right now, and which could use adjustment?

What one small action could I take this week to support my physical, emotional, or mental well-being?

How can I celebrate the progress I've already made, even if it feels incremental?

Tip: Review and Reflect Weekly

Set aside a few minutes at the end of each week to review your symptom checklist and reflection answers. Look for patterns, celebrate small wins, and note any shifts in how you feel physically, emotionally, and mentally. This practice helps you spot trends, adjust strategies, and reinforce your sense of agency as you navigate perimenopause.

Final Thoughts

Now that you understand what perimenopause really is beyond the myths and shame, you can start to see it as a chance to pause, listen, and care for yourself in new ways. Recognizing the physical and emotional shifts as natural signals allows you to respond with curiosity instead of fear, building habits that support your well-being today and in the future.

This phase invites you to reset priorities, adjust routines, and strengthen self-trust so you feel more grounded and ready for the changes ahead. With clear information and compassionate self-awareness, you can change your perception of perimenopause from a time of loss to an opportunity to shape how you live, work, and thrive in the years to come.

Chapter 2:

Hormones and the Body-Brain Connection—How Fluctuations Drive Mood, Sleep, Appetite, and Metabolism

How many times a day do you notice your mood shifting for no clear reason, or find yourself unable to fall asleep even when you're exhausted? Maybe your appetite plays tricks on you: one moment you feel full, and the next, you're craving all kinds of comfort food. If you've found yourself wondering what's behind these sudden shifts, you're not alone.

These are the subtle, and sometimes not-so-subtle, signals your hormones are sending back and forth between your body and brain. Understanding these messages can feel like unlocking a new level of self-awareness. It gives you the power to see your experiences in a new light. You begin to realize it's less about what's wrong with you and more about what's happening inside your body.

Let's explore those hormonal ups, downs, and everything in between, and how they influence not only how you feel but also how you rest, eat, and move through your day. This is about meeting this phase with knowledge and kindness, turning what feels unpredictable into manageable moments.

Hormones and Their Impact on Mood, Cognition, and Emotional Regulation

Many different hormones are involved in perimenopause, and understanding how they work both together and against each other is an important step in making the necessary changes to reset your life.

Let's start with estrogen, one of the most important hormones for your reproductive health. Estrogen is at the center of hormonal changes during perimenopause. It influences almost every system in your body, from your reproductive organs to your brain and metabolism.

This is why estrogen is often called the "master regulator." It doesn't just control your menstrual cycle and fertility, but also shapes how your brain feels, thinks, and responds to the world (Nichols, 2025). This all changes during perimenopause. Instead of steadily dropping as it did during regular monthly cycles, it rises and falls in unpredictable surges. This means that one week, you might have a heavy period and feel strangely energized, then a few days later experience hot flashes, mood dips, and even trouble sleeping.

Estrogen also helps regulate neurotransmitters, such as serotonin and dopamine. These brain chemicals help to control your mood, appetite, and even sleep (Bendis et al., 2024). When your estrogen is high, you'll feel upbeat, clear-headed, and sociable. But when it plummets, the opposite can happen. You may become irritable, feel anxious, and your appetite may spike or drop suddenly, and cravings for sugary or salty foods can become intense. During these times, it's common to wonder, "Why does my mood change so quickly?" or "Why do I suddenly crave chips at midnight?"

In the early stages of estrogen's unpredictable dance, progesterone brings a dose of calm. As perimenopause starts, your progesterone begins to decline before estrogen does. But unlike estrogen, which fluctuates drastically at times, your progesterone levels decline steadily over time (*Progesterone Changes in Perimenopause*, 2024). Healthy levels of progesterone soothe your brain and your nervous system. It helps you feel steady, less anxious, and more able to sleep peacefully. For many years, this hormone has served as an emotional cushion, helping you deal with stress, irritability, and frustration.

When your progesterone levels drop, those calming effects weaken. Your body's built-in brake on anxiety and sleeplessness is gone, making it much easier to feel jumpy, short-tempered, or tossed around by racing thoughts at night. Your sleep patterns might change dramatically. You may toss and turn for hours before you finally drift off, or perhaps you may fall asleep easily, but wake up at 3 a.m. with a restless mind. During the day, you might snap at people over small things that wouldn't normally even bother you. It's not due to a lack of willpower or a personal flaw. Your nervous system has lost part of its natural buffer.

Then there's cortisol, the stress hormone, that increases when you respond to stress. It's produced by the adrenal glands, and helps your body respond quickly to challenges, giving a burst of energy or focus when needed (Woods et al., 2009). When your cortisol level is too high or out of rhythm, you'll struggle to cope with life's challenges even more. During perimenopause, the fluctuations in estrogen and progesterone can disrupt the way your brain (specifically the hypothalamus and pituitary gland) coordinates with the adrenal glands. This results in your cortisol peaking at the wrong moments or remaining elevated for longer stretches.

When your cortisol spikes while your progesterone is low and your estrogen is unstable, the effects will feel magnified. You'll likely feel tired more often, struggle more with mood swings and cravings, and many other typical challenges of perimenopause will feel out of control.

How Hormones Interact and Create Daily Swings

Your estrogen, progesterone, and cortisol aren't operating in separate worlds. A shift in one of these hormones triggers changes in the others. When your estrogen surges or drops, it affects the way your brain responds to stress. If your progesterone is low during an estrogen swing, your nervous system loses the ability to stay calm, so stress hits harder. In periods when your cortisol is already high from poor sleep, pressure at work, or family crises, the combined effects can add up quickly (Edwards & Mills, 2008). You'll struggle to sleep, have more mood dips, and simple decisions might suddenly seem overwhelming.

This cycle of rising and falling hormones, and their ongoing conversations with one another, explains why your day-to-day experiences can feel so different. One morning, the world may seem bright and full of possibility. The next morning, you may feel anxious, foggy, or on the edge of tears. Noticing these patterns for what they are will help you understand that your symptoms are responses to changing chemistry, not a failing of your character or effort.

Awareness allows you to anticipate tougher days, pace yourself, and respond with gentle, practical strategies.

Your Hormones' Effect on Appetite, Cravings, and Your Metabolism

Now that you understand how the hormones affected by perimenopause can impact your mood, cognitive function, and emotions, you may wonder why they can also make you want to reach for a snack even when you've just had a meal. The answer is quite simple: Your hormones tell your brain when it's time to eat and also what type of food your body needs. When your hormonal levels are fluctuating, as is the case during perimenopause, they send mixed messages. One day, you may feel satisfied after eating an omelet. Another, you may experience a hunger that shows up out of nowhere by mid-afternoon, stubborn and sharp, even after a good lunch.

Fluctuating estrogen and progesterone play a central role in these sudden shifts. Higher estrogen tends to keep your hunger at bay and make it easier to notice when you're full. When your estrogen dips, your appetite can increase, and you may find yourself having unusual cravings (Hirschberg, 2012). The desire for comfort foods, such as pizza, bread, crackers, or chocolate, isn't random or due to a lack of discipline. It's your body picking up on hormone cues.

Progesterone has its own influence. When it falls, your brain gets fuzzy, and the gut slows down, making it harder to notice those natural "I'm full" signals. That is why you may feel hungry shortly after finishing a meal.

These changes in your appetite and cravings are directly linked to your hormones and emotions. Your monthly cycle, including your follicular phase, ovulation, and premenstrual swings, affects how full or hungry you feel. This is deeply tied to serotonin production in your brain. Serotonin is a hormone that affects your mood, sleep, digestion, and many other bodily functions. When your estrogen level drops, your body will also produce less serotonin. As a result, your body will crave carbs and sugar, as these are two quick ways to give your brain a mood boost (Scaccia, 2022).

Building Trust With Cravings

When your appetite changes and weird cravings take over, responding with curiosity instead of guilt can be a game-changer. Intuitive eating means tuning in to these signals without harsh judgment. This means asking yourself questions to understand the real reason for these changes in your eating habits. For example, you can ask yourself, "Is the craving a way to self-soothe after a tough meeting, or do I have other symptoms to suggest my hormones are fluctuating?" Once you understand the reason, you can manage it. For example, giving yourself permission to eat a limited amount of certain foods, rather than restricting them altogether, takes away their power. Over time, this builds a relationship of trust rather than friction with food choices.

On top of hunger and cravings, perimenopause changes how your body breaks down and stores energy. With age, your metabolism naturally slows. On top of this, lower estrogen makes your body less sensitive to insulin, changing how efficiently it uses glucose for energy. This can lead to blood sugar swings, stronger hunger signals, and, for many, easier fat storage. This excess in fat storage is often around your abdomen.

Progesterone also affects your digestion. Lower levels mean slower gut movement, leading to feelings of bloating or fullness that last longer. This can make it harder to figure out if your body really needs food, or if it just feels "off." All of these changes can be frustrating, especially if your clothes fit differently or the number on the scale creeps up. But these shifts are normal responses to a changing biological landscape. In Chapter 5, we'll discuss eating habits during perimenopause, as well as simple strategies to help you take ownership of your body during this time of transition.

Why Hormones Can Cause Sleepless Nights

During perimenopause, fluctuating hormone levels can have a big impact on your sleep patterns. As progesterone drops, your body loses a natural calming, sleep-promoting hormone that usually encourages deep, restorative rest and soothes your nervous system. With lower progesterone levels, you may find yourself waking frequently or too early, struggling to return to sleep, or sleeping lightly without feeling refreshed.

Lower levels of estrogen add to these disturbances by disrupting your body's temperature regulation (Haufe & Leeners, 2023). This can lead to nighttime hot flashes and night sweats, including sudden heat surges that interrupt your sleep and cause repeated awakenings, further affecting your rest. These hormonal shifts can make bedtime feel daunting as you may anticipate another restless night, before you even get into bed.

The production of melatonin, the hormone that signals to your brain when it's time to rest, is also disrupted during perimenopause (*Melatonin*, 2025). Estrogen and progesterone influence melatonin's production and timing, so when they decrease, your sleep windows shift earlier or later, or make it more difficult to fall and stay asleep. External factors such as stress, shift work, travel, and screen time further add to this, causing unpredictable bedtimes and fragmented sleep.

Poor sleep during perimenopause goes beyond fatigue. It impairs your cognitive functions, including slower reaction times, memory challenges, and reduced patience, and negatively affects mood, often creating feelings of anxiety, irritability, or flatness (Watson & Cherney, 2025). Additionally, tired brains crave quick energy sources, leading to increased appetite for sweets, caffeine, or comfort foods. This creates a feedback loop: Disrupted sleep misaligns your hunger cues, disturbs blood sugar and appetite, and subsequently worsens your sleep patterns.

Translating Hormonal Understanding Into Daily Choices

During perimenopause, your hormones are shifting, and these changes ripple through your body, mind, and emotions. While these fluctuations can feel unpredictable or overwhelming, learning to track your symptoms, moods, appetite, and sleep can transform uncertainty into clarity.

By observing your unique patterns, you can anticipate challenging days, adjust habits mindfully, and make compassionate choices that support your well-being. Tracking is an extremely helpful tool for understanding yourself, guiding your decisions, and treating yourself with kindness during this transformative phase.

Use the activities and reflection prompts in this section to build awareness, develop supportive routines, and honor both your body and mind.

Create Your Own Tracker

You can use a simple notebook, planner, or a phone app, whatever feels easiest and most sustainable for you. The goal is just to get to know yourself and your body better so you can understand your mood, energy, and cravings so you can make informed, compassionate choices for your reset.

Category	**What to track**
Physical symptoms	Hot flashes, headaches, bloating, cravings, or other changes
Mood	Times when emotions feel intense, low, or unsteady

Appetite	When and what you feel hungry for; note cravings too
Sleep	Hours slept and how rested you feel upon waking

Reflection questions:

What patterns do I notice? Are there days with more symptoms or mood shifts?

____

____

____

____

____

How do these patterns affect my daily energy or choices?

____

____

____

____

____

What self-compassionate reminders can I give myself when symptoms feel tough?

____

____

____

____

____

____

Notice Your Habits, Appetite, and Cravings

Perimenopause can bring changes in appetite, digestion, and cravings, often influenced by shifting hormones. Instead of following rigid rules, a flexible, mindful approach to eating helps you observe your habits, tune into your body's needs, and reduce stress or guilt around food.

Before your next meal or snack, take a few intentional moments to check in. This exercise helps you notice your eating habits, appetite changes, and cravings, so you can make choices that feel nourishing and satisfying.

Pause and Ask Questions

Before you eat, stop and take a deep breath. Give yourself a moment to check in with your body and mind. Then ask yourself: Am I physically hungry, or is this hunger emotional, habitual, or triggered by a routine or craving?

- **Physical hunger:** builds gradually and feels satisfied by nutritious food
- **Emotional or habitual hunger:** feels urgent, tied to stress, boredom, or routine

My answer today:

____

____

____

___

___

___

Notice Your Eating Habits and Cravings Without Judgment

Pay attention to what type of food you're craving, why you're eating, and any cravings that arise.

Habits and cravings I notice:

___

___

___

___

___

Sleep Routine Checklist

Build a wind-down routine that helps signal to your body it's time for rest. Check off each step as you do it:

- ▢ consistent bedtime and wake-up time
- ▢ dimming lights and turning off screens 30–60 minutes before bed
- ▢ relaxing activity (for example, reading, taking a warm shower, or drinking herbal tea)

My wind-down routine tonight:

After you wake up the next morning, reflect: How did I sleep the previous night?

Use your daily tracker and reflections to notice patterns and gain insight into your body's hormonal rhythms. Let this awareness guide your choices with compassion, flexibility, and mindfulness. Over time, these practices create a foundation of balance, supporting your well-being through perimenopause and beyond.

Final Thoughts

Now that you understand how perimenopause shifts hormones that affect your mood, sleep, appetite, and energy, stop blaming yourself for these unpredictable changes. Recognizing these symptoms as natural responses to hormonal patterns opens the door for you to be kind to yourself and take practical action. With this awareness, you gain the tools to track your unique rhythms, gently adjust your daily habits, and create space for rest and self-care without adding pressure.

By doing this, you start a reset that supports your body and mind through these transitions, laying a strong foundation for greater ease and well-being as you move toward menopause.

Chapter 3:

Identity, Body Image, and Self-Worth in Transition

What happens when the reflection in the mirror no longer matches the woman you've always known? How do you make sense of a body that feels less familiar, while your inner voice grows louder with doubts and questions about who you are now? If you've noticed shifts in your energy, mood, or how you see yourself, you're not alone.

These changes can cause a lot of discomfort, but if you choose to approach this phase of life with curiosity, you can challenge long-held beliefs about worth tied to appearance and youth. Let's discuss those questions that may be making you feel uneasy with kindness and an open mind, and explore how this transformation can reveal new ways to value yourself during this unique time.

Society, Messaging, and Self-Worth

When you walk through any magazine aisle, scroll through social media, or turn on the television, you'll see the same story repeating itself. Images of fresh faces, smooth skin, and youthful bodies are everywhere. Clothing brands, beauty ads, and popular movies often choose youth as their standard for what is beautiful, energetic, or valuable. This isn't just in the background. It filters into daily conversations, workplace expectations, and even the doctor's offices. Wrinkles, gray hair, sagging skin, hot flashes, all typical signals of perimenopause, clash with notions that youth equals worthiness.

These cultural scripts work in quiet but powerful ways. Every day, language makes you think about aging as something to battle, reverse, or hide. Birthday cards joke about being "over the hill." Beauty products promise to "erase the signs of aging." Compliments often sound something like, "You look so young for your age," as if it's a sign of success. During perimenopause, when changes like weight shifts or thinning hair become visible, you may feel even more pressure to maintain a youthful look. The fear of "losing" value creeps in as each subtle shift stands out against these ideals.

This tension spills into your self-esteem and body image. When society keeps telling you that being young and flawless makes you desirable, your self-doubt grows every time you notice changes in the mirror. You might try to hide your gray hair or feel embarrassed about hot flashes at work, even though these are completely normal and shared experiences. The shame, guilt, or anxiety you feel comes from being measured against an impossible expectation.

Even if these beliefs only start to really bother you in midlife, they've been building for years, slowly changing the way you talk to yourself inside your head. Commercials for anti-wrinkle creams, offhand comments from friends or partners, and unspoken rules about how women "should" age all sneak into your internal script. Over time, that critical voice saying "You look tired" or "You're not attractive anymore" starts to sound more like you than anyone else.

- "If my body doesn't look the way it did in my 20s, I'm less valuable."
- "Visible signs of aging mean I'm past my prime."
- "Menopause makes me invisible or irrelevant."
- "I need to apologize for my appearance."

These judgments change how you move through the world. You might skip social events, avoid mirrors, or cover yourself in ways that don't feel comfortable, all in an effort to escape shame. You may also find yourself over-investing in products or procedures that promise a return to youth, even when these solutions never feel truly satisfying. By recognizing these habits in yourself, you begin to see how much your inner dialogue is shaped by years of exposure to unrealistic external standards.

Social media and mass marketing only make this worse. Perfectly edited selfies, filters that erase wrinkles, and influencer posts praising quick fixes all reinforce the fantasy that aging can be paused or reversed with the right choices. As you scroll through these images, it's easy to compare your unfiltered reality to a highlight reel created through filters and editing. Suddenly, ordinary changes like belly fat, hair texture, or skin spots feel wrong or shameful, even though they are completely natural.

Finding self-worth beyond appearance is an ongoing practice for you. It starts with curiosity about where your beliefs took root and continues with the steady work of noticing and questioning self-critical thoughts. Spaces that share the real stories of perimenopause can help quiet those old voices and invite new ones into your life. This awareness opens the door for you to examine your personal beliefs and develop a more supportive self-dialogue, ready for deeper exploration.

Navigating Physical and Identity Changes

What makes these ideals from society and the media about how you "ought" to look or act even more challenging to deal with is that they tend to stick. Over time, these messages often become automatic beliefs that change the way you see yourself, especially during perimenopause.

The first step in shifting these internal narratives is to notice them as they happen. Automatic thoughts are knee-jerk reactions in your mind. They pop up so quickly that you might not realize they're there. For example, if you see gray hair or new wrinkles, your mind might flash the message, "I look so old". These are automatic thoughts and instant judgments, not truths. Being able to notice and accept these moments for what they truly are is both a skill and a form of self-care.

One way to do this is by making a quick mental note each time you catch an unrealistic or overly critical thought. You might find it easier to jot them down. A journal kept on your phone or in a notebook can help you spot repeating patterns. Write down exactly what you thought in the moment, without editing. For instance, "I hate the way my arms look in short sleeves" or "No one will find me attractive now." Collecting these for a few days often reveals previously invisible patterns. Remember, this isn't about scolding yourself, but rather about gathering information gently. The simple act of labeling a thought as "just a thought" can lessen its sting.

After you've identified some of your automatic thoughts, the next step is to challenge what your brain is telling you. Many automatic thoughts are shaped by cognitive distortions, which are mental habits that warp reality and reinforce negative self-views. Understanding these can make them easier to question.

Emma's Story: Navigating Identity in Perimenopause

Emma (44) has always defined herself by being active, energetic, and in control of her appearance. Over the past year, she's noticed weight shifts, thinning hair, and low energy. Stress and hormonal changes sometimes trigger emotional eating, leaving her feeling guilty, frustrated, and disconnected from herself.

She began journaling her automatic thoughts and behaviors, noticing a cycle: a critical thought turned into skipping exercise or overeating, which led to shame and reinforcing negative beliefs about her body. By mapping these patterns, Emma realized her beliefs weren't facts. They were assumptions she could challenge.

Emma started reframing her thoughts: Instead of "I'm too tired to exercise," she tried, "My energy is different today, and a short walk still supports my health." She paired these thoughts with small, values-driven actions, like walking with a friend or taking a mindful pause. Over time, these gentle experiments helped her rebuild self-compassion, reconnect with her body, and create habits aligned with her values rather than appearance.

Common Cognitive Distortions

Just like Emma recognized her own negative thoughts, you can become aware of the automatic thoughts you might have. Let's look at a few common cognitive distortions that many women struggle with during perimenopause, and how you can challenge them:

- **Catastrophizing:** Jumping to the worst possible outcome.
  - Example: "If my body is changing, I'll never feel good about myself again."
  - Challenge this thought: "Is it true I'll never feel good again? Have there been times recently when I've felt good about myself? What makes me doubt myself?"
- **All-or-nothing thinking:** Seeing situations in black-and-white, with no middle ground.
  - Example: "If I'm not as thin as I was, I'm unattractive."
  - Challenge this thought: "Can I be attractive in ways that don't depend on my size? Have others valued different qualities in me?"
- **Overgeneralization:** Drawing sweeping judgments from single events.
  - Example: "I look terrible in photos. I don't ever want any photos taken of myself."
  - Challenge this thought: "Does one bad picture mean I never look good in any photo? Have I liked recent photos of myself?"

- **Mental filtering:** Focusing only on flaws and ignoring strengths or positives.
    - Example: "All I see are my wrinkles."
    - Challenge this thought: "What about my laugh lines, or how expressive my face is when I smile? Is that not a sign that I have had good experiences in my life?"

Challenging these patterns can feel like detective work. Ask yourself: "Is this thought completely true?" or "What would I say to a close friend if I heard her say this?" The more you question these thoughts and limiting beliefs, the more you'll come to realize that they aren't based on facts.

Reframe Your Negative Thoughts

The process doesn't end at challenging your negative thoughts and limiting beliefs. Once you've identified them, replace them with fresh, compassionate ones. Cognitive reframing is about landing on more accurate and kind alternatives, rather than pretending that everything's perfect. Take the thought, "I'll never be attractive again." A reframed version might sound like, "My appearance is changing, and I'm finding new qualities in myself." Turning "My body is failing me" into "My body is adapting, and I'm learning different ways to care for it," acknowledges this change while opening space for new strengths. This step means treating your thoughts as hypotheses rather than hard facts.

Next, anchor these new beliefs to an experience. When you act "as if" the kinder thought is true, your behavior and the evidence you gather can reshape your mind and what you believe. This is where behavioral experiments come in. These are small, practical tests to see whether your negative beliefs hold up compared to your newly reframed thought.

Try a self-care routine that honors your changing body, like using scented lotion or taking a walk. While you do this, repeat a positive phrase you want to believe. Notice how your body feels and how your mood changes. Or, if you've been feeling invisible, make eye contact or start up a short conversation with a cashier or coworker. Pay attention to the actual response. Wear something that feels like an authentic reflection of who you are now, rather than what you "should" wear, and see how you feel.

Each small experiment creates new data. If the outcome goes better than expected, you start building a mental library of counterexamples to old negative beliefs. These lived experiences help your brain register that other outcomes are possible. Over time, these experiments encourage a more balanced, grounded view and remind you to treat yourself with kindness as you learn and grow through change.

Cognitive Reframing for a Positive Self-View

Catching a critical thought and reframing it with a positive one is a big win, but actually treating yourself with kindness takes a little more. The work you did with cognitive reframing helps you spot old habits, like seeing a new curve or a bad mood, and instead of instantly blaming yourself, accept them for what they are. Still, spotting unhelpful thoughts only solves part of the puzzle. The other side is learning how to respond when difficulty shows up. That response is the heart of self-compassion: not in challenging what you think, but in changing how you support yourself through it.

Self-compassion is a practice you can learn, no matter how tough you've been on yourself in the past. Think of how you'd comfort a close friend who is struggling. You'll likely treat them with warmth and encouragement without expecting them to just "snap out of it." That same steady kindness belongs to you, too. You're not looking for excuses or letting yourself off the hook. Scientific studies show that self-compassion actually lowers shame, builds resilience, and helps you grow during tough changes (Cepni et al., 2024). At the same time, it keeps you honest about what's really hard, without beating yourself up for it.

Three main ideas make up self-compassion.

- **Mindfulness:** This practice is about noticing what you feel and think without denying it or making it bigger than it is. For example, if you catch yourself thinking, "I hate how my body looks," mindfulness allows you to notice the thought as just that: a thought. By doing this, you accept the thought without ignoring it or letting it take over. This pause makes room for a gentler response and steers you away from that familiar cycle of shame or criticism.

- **Humanity:** Going through changes that make you feel sad, frustrated, or out of sorts is by no means a sign of personal failure. Every woman moving through perimenopause feels some of this, and sometimes a lot of it. Remembering you aren't alone stops the suffering from doubling back on itself. You replace "What's wrong with me?" with "This is human. Other women feel this too." Even naming the shared struggle can bring a little relief and a sense of connection.

- **Self-kindness:** Most of the time, self-talk slips into a harsher tone than you'd use when talking to anyone else. Facing vulnerability brings out criticism, for example, "I'm losing everything that made me attractive." Trying self-kindness in that moment sounds like, "My body's changing, and that hurts. But my body still carries me through each day and hasn't given up on me." When you mess up or fall short, for example, missing a workout, or snapping at a loved one, the critical line might be, "I should be handling this better." A kind reply is, "This is hard for a lot of women. I'm trying with what I've got right now." Your words don't have to be unrealistically cheerful. Small shifts signal to your brain that you're someone worth caring for, even when you don't have all the answers.

The more often you bring compassion to yourself, the more it influences what you do next. Maybe you let yourself rest one day instead of pushing through exhaustion, or perhaps you learn to disregard a thought that isn't serving you. The way you speak shapes what you choose, and the more you do this, the more you'll see that connection showing up in your habits, too.

Here are two simple ways to build self-compassion into your daily life.

Self-Compassion Letter Writing

1. Find a quiet moment. About 15 to 20 minutes will do. Have a pen and paper ready, or open a document where you can type.

2. Pick a struggle related to perimenopause, for example, a body change, tough emotion, or shift in identity. Write it down in a sentence or two.

3. Imagine a dear friend sharing the same struggle. What would you say to her? Write it down, letting your empathy and warmth show up, without holding back.

4. Next, write a letter to yourself about your own struggle, using those same caring words you would use when talking to a friend.

5. Read your letter aloud. Notice what feelings or pushback come up. Curiosity is enough here.

6. Keep the letter close, and reread it when you need support, especially on tough days.

Compassionate Touch Meditation

1. Sit or lie down comfortably. Close your eyes or soften your gaze.

2. Think of something you're struggling with. Notice any tension or discomfort in your body.

3. Gently place your hands on your heart, belly, or face, wherever feels most comforting.

4. Feel the warmth and steady rhythm of your breath under your hands.

5. Silently repeat soft phrases such as "I may be kind to myself," or "I may accept myself as I am."

6. Continue for a few minutes, letting the touch and phrases work together.

7. When you're done, breathe deeply and check in with how you feel.

Both of these practices help activate your body's calming system and teach your brain a new way to respond, building the habit of kindness. Doing something short every day matters much more than making it perfect or long.

You might doubt whether self-compassion will work or worry that it makes change harder. The opposite is true: treating yourself kindly lowers harshness and actually keeps you moving, rather than getting stuck in shame.

It's normal for you to feel awkward or even fake when you treat yourself with kindness. That comes from years of self-criticism, but practice makes it familiar. Over time, compassion becomes a resource you can reach for no matter where you are in your journey.

Self-Compassion and Linking Identity to Daily Habits

Identity and daily habits are partners in a silent dance. Each shift in how you see yourself reveals itself in how you use your body, your energy, and your time. It's natural for old patterns to suddenly feel out of reach when perimenopause changes the way you feel in your skin. You might have seen exercise as something you did because you were strong and liked the challenge, but doubts about energy or changes in your body may start to whisper that you no longer belong in that world. Sometimes food turns from a way to nourish yourself into a battleground because a changing middle or stubborn bloating stirs up the old belief that being thin means you're worthy.

Habits are often shaped by your thoughts. If you wake up thinking, "My body is unpredictable. I can't rely on it," you're less likely to lace up your shoes for a walk or reach for a healthy breakfast. The habit of skipping meals or eating in secret often has little to do with hunger and much to do with lingering guilt or fear that controlling food is the same as controlling your life. The patterns may slip in unannounced: avoiding social gatherings because you don't feel beautiful, hitting snooze again because your energy is low, or overbooking your calendar in an effort to push aside uncomfortable feelings of change.

Noticing this link between your inner stories and outer actions is where the first puzzle piece clicks. When you change your story, even a little, you create the chance to choose differently. There's a world of difference between thinking "I'm not good enough to join that fitness class" and "My energy is changing, so I'll try something new that matches where I am." That opening creates room for fresh habits, ones that build you up rather than break you down.

Values help anchor your new habits. Unlike goals, which are destinations to reach, values are like a compass that keeps pointing in the same direction no matter where you stand. Ask yourself what you want your life to stand for as your identity evolves. Do you want to honor health over appearance? Is connection with others, or with yourself, at the center? Does joy matter more than appearance? Clarity here makes everything simpler. When you know your true north, you can say "yes" to what supports it and "no" to the noise of culture or old expectations.

Let's look at a few examples. Instead of forcing yourself into a punishing workout because you feel like that is what you "should" do, you might take a walk outdoors with a friend because friendship and movement both matter. By doing this, you remove the pressure of working out and instead do something that goes with your energy and fits in your life. Eating something colorful and satisfying at lunch can shift from a duty to self-control to an act of self-respect. Rest might become a way to honor your body's needs, rather than a sign that you're lazy or giving up.

These values-driven habits are most sustainable when you spot and interrupt the cycles that keep you stuck. There are moments when old, negative thoughts, such as *I don't belong anymore*, *I'm invisible*, or *I'm never going to feel comfortable in my body again*, resurface and, with that, an old habit rushes in to fix or numb that feeling. Maybe you restrict food too much, over-exercise, withdraw from others, or stay up late scrolling through your phone. These are more than just habits. They're the mind's way of trying to feel safe again, even if the comfort is fleeting.

Take a moment to picture this cycle: You believe you're too self-conscious to join an outing, so you cancel. Later, you feel isolated. That only confirms the belief that you don't fit in. The key here is to see this chain without judgment. Instead, use this moment to become curious. Ask yourself, "What am I hoping this habit will do for me right now? What pain am I trying to soothe?" Start to notice the trigger: the thought or feeling that sets things in motion.

One gentle way forward is to create new, small rituals that say, "I matter as I am." It doesn't have to be a big effort. Smaller acts of kindness toward yourself are easier to continue with and add up over time. A five-minute stretching routine that feels good, not punishing, can be repeated daily. Try a single meal each day without distractions, noticing the taste, feel, and effect of the food you choose. Schedule 30 minutes in your week for something that reinforces a valued part of yourself, such as painting, reading, calling a friend, or tending to your plants. These modest changes are doable and give you regular reminders that care and self-worth are available, no matter what your body or mood is that day. Over time, these actions reshape how you see yourself far more than any dramatic overhaul could.

Behavioral Pattern Map Worksheet

Let's look at two exercises to help you change the way you view yourself during perimenopause. Use this worksheet to map out the connection between your identity beliefs and your daily habits. It helps you spot cycles and opens space for new choices.

List a recurring negative thought or belief about myself (for example: "I'm not strong anymore").

___

___

___

Write down the specific situation when this belief usually shows up.

Describe the habit or behavior that follows, such as skipping a workout, overeating, or isolating yourself.

Notice the outcome: How do I feel afterwards? What effect does it have on my self-perception?

Next to this, brainstorm one alternative action that could disrupt the cycle, even if it's something small.

Try this new action the next time the situation arises and record how it felt. Review your notes at the end of the week and look for any shifts in feelings or beliefs.

Reflection Prompts for Positive Self-Talk and Self-Worth

Try these prompts to replace harsh self-talk with kinder, more helpful thoughts that support evolving self-worth.

Name one thing my body allows me to experience or enjoy today.

Write down a recent habit I feel proud of, no matter how tiny.

If I catch a critical thought, pause and ask: "Would I say this to a close friend?"

List three qualities that matter to me beyond appearance. Examples of this can include creativity, patience, or kindness.

1. ______________________________

____

____

2. ______________________________

____

____

3. ______________________________

____

____

At the end of the day, jot down one way I honored my values through any small choice or action.

____

____

____

____

____

____

____

____

____

Final Thoughts

Now that you've explored how perimenopause reshapes your body as well as your sense of self, you can begin to turn those uneasy feelings into opportunities for growth. By noticing the stories you tell yourself and gently challenging old beliefs, you open the door to greater self-compassion and renewed confidence. Using tools like the behavioral pattern map to track habits and reflection prompts to build kinder self-talk helps you create new routines that honor who you are today.

End of Week 2 Reflection and Reset Check-In

As you complete the first two weeks of your perimenopause reset journey, this reflection and reset check-in invites you to pause and integrate your learning so far. Use this space to connect insights from your physical symptoms, emotional shifts, and changing mindset. By reviewing patterns and deepening your self-awareness, you'll build a stronger foundation for compassionate, intentional change. This is your opportunity to honor progress, understand challenges, and set gentle goals that support your unique path forward.

Synthesizing Your Experiences

Think broadly about the physical, emotional, and cognitive changes you've tracked and noticed. Use these prompts to connect the dots:

Which new insights about perimenopause surprised or stood out to me most during these weeks?

____

____

____

____

____

____

____

____

____

____

How have my physical symptoms, emotions, and thoughts seemed to interact or influence each other?

I remember a moment when understanding my hormonal changes helped shift my perspective and response. What happened and how?

Exploring Your Relationship with Change

Perimenopause is as much about identity and mindset as it is about biology. Explore your evolving relationship with yourself:

How am I feeling about the personal changes perimenopause is bringing? This can include acceptance, frustration, and curiosity.

What internalized beliefs or messages about aging or worth surfaced for me during these weeks?

What new self-compassion practices or thoughts have I found helpful or want to try?

____

____

____

____

____

____

____

____

Identifying Patterns and Triggers

Review your notes or trackers from the past two weeks and reflect on what you observe:

Are there specific times, situations, or activities that tend to worsen or improve my symptoms or mood?

____

____

____

____

____

____

____

What signs or "red flags" have I learned to recognize indicating a need for extra care or rest?

How do my habits align with these patterns? What feels supportive or misaligned? This can include eating, movement, and sleep patterns.

Setting Priorities and Gentle Goals

Based on your reflections, create two to three small, achievable intentions that honor your current state and goals:

Physical goal (for example, prioritize restful sleep, or manage a specific symptom):

____

____

____

____

____

Emotional/mindset goal (for example, practice a daily kindness ritual or challenge negative self-talk):

____

____

____

____

____

Behavioral goal (for example, commit to mindful eating once daily or try a new gentle movement):

____

____

____

____

Planning for Support and Continued Growth

Sustaining change requires compassion and flexibility. Use these prompts to prepare your mindset and environment:

What support systems can I lean on or develop? This can include family, friends, trained professionals, or other resources.

____

____

____

____

____

____

____

How will I remind myself to practice patience and kindness in moments of struggle?

____

____

____

____

____

____

____

____

What phrase, image, or personal mantra could inspire me to keep going on challenging days?

____

____

____

____

____

Final Reflection: Your Reset Check-In

Write a brief message to myself about where I am now in this reset journey and what I hope to carry forward:

____

____

____

____

Remember, this reset is a journey, not a race. Use this reflection regularly to stay connected with your body and mind, adjusting your habits with kindness and flexibility as you go. Embrace each insight as a step toward greater balance and resilience. You're not just creating new routines, but a renewed relationship with yourself through perimenopause and beyond. Keep nurturing this connection. You have everything you need to thrive.

Part II:

Foundational Reset

(Weeks 3 to 4)

Chapter 4:

The Six Pillars in Practice. Building a Balanced Lifestyle that Supports Hormonal Health

The late afternoon sun filters softly through the kitchen window as you reach for yet another cup of coffee, your thoughts already tangled in the demands of meetings, errands, and the ever-growing to-do list. A familiar tension gathers in your shoulders, and the restless energy that has been simmering beneath the surface all week begins to chip away at your sense of calm. You sense something shifting, not just the usual busyness, but a deeper, quieter current pulling at your balance and well-being. How often do you find yourself feeling this way, as if everything is moving faster inside than the world around you? Or have you noticed subtle changes in your energy, mood, or clarity that you can't quite put into words yet?

In these moments, small choices start to carry outsized weight. What you eat, how you move, when you choose to pause or breathe are gentle acts that become the anchors that steady your days. They're not quick fixes or rigid rules imposed from outside but personal invitations to nurture yourself amid change.

Let's look at those six pillars—eating, movement, stress, sleep, emotions, and imbalances—that work together to build a resilient, balanced foundation. Here, you'll discover practical ways to turn intention into action, creating steady ground beneath your feet even when everything else feels unsettled.

Finding Your Ground: Why the Six Pillars Matter Now

Perimenopause can feel like a wild ride with no warning signs or a clear map. The one minute, you're energized, feeling sharp, and flowing through your day. The next minute, fog descends, leaving you exhausted and struggling to manage mood swings that feel both sudden and overwhelming. Your body and mind pulse with change, both on the surface and also deep within, where fluctuating hormones break the former predictable rhythms of your cells, tissues, and brain chemistry. Without steady anchors, this shifting landscape can leave you unsure of yourself, creating a sense of imbalance that changes everything from how you relate to others to how you see yourself.

Imagine moving through each day without clear landmarks. Your energy may spike and crash without reason or foresight. Sleep might fragment, leaving you tired but wired. Cravings can hijack your intentions, and emotions intensify like waves you can neither predict nor ride out. Without support, these fluctuations threaten your daily life and your long-term health.

Now, picture what happens if your struggles continue unchecked into menopause itself. The hormonal shifts of menopause often amplify your earlier perimenopausal symptoms, but when it's compounded by years of disorganized habits, unmanaged stress, and disrupted sleep, you may face intensified hot flashes, weight gain, bone loss, cognitive fog, and emotional distress. The absence of foundational lifestyle practices can make this transition feel heavier, more isolating, and more challenging to navigate. In contrast, if you develop stability during perimenopause, you're likely to experience a smoother menopause, with less severe symptoms and greater resilience.

This is why perimenopause is so much more than just a natural period of change. It's a precious window of opportunity to reset. It allows you to press pause, build strength, and build habits that serve you both now and down the road. At the heart of this reset lies six interconnected lifestyle pillars: eating, movement, stress, sleep, emotions, and imbalances.

Think of these six pillars as strong yet flexible supports holding up the structure of your health, mental health and well-being during this phase. Each pillar shapes your experience in unique ways, but together they create a harmonious system that helps your body and mind adapt with grace, steadiness, and strength as your hormones fluctuate.

These pillars don't exist in isolation. Rather, they engage in a dynamic balance of cause and effect. For example, improving your sleep supports steadier moods and better appetite regulation. Regular movement enhances your energy levels and makes it easier to rest peacefully. Managing stress reduces cravings and improves emotional balance. When you nurture one pillar, the others often respond and rise with it, creating an upward rhythm toward greater wellness.

This chapter serves as your guide to understanding these pillars in depth. It will help you weave small, intentional habits into your daily life to honor your individuality and busy schedule. These practices are invitations to meet perimenopause with compassion, curiosity, and strength. By seeing these six pillars as your anchors, you're building a foundation that holds steady amid change.

With this groundwork in place, you'll be better equipped to face the unpredictable rhythms of perimenopause and prepare for a lighter, more balanced transition into the years ahead.

Pillar One: Eating (with Awareness and Intuition)

When it comes to perimenopause, what you eat matters more than ever. Your body is going through a bunch of changes, and those hormone shifts affect everything from how your metabolism works to when and what you feel hungry for. That afternoon snack craving or feeling hungry again right after you eat is more than likely emotional eating and hormones wreaking havoc in your body.

So, the goal here isn't about strict diets or counting every calorie, but rather about steady, reliable nourishment that helps supports hormone balance, and keeps your emotions stable. Feeding your body well means fueling yourself with kindness and practicality so you can feel stronger and more in control through this phase.

Protein: Your Hormone's Best Friend

Protein is one of the most important pieces of the puzzle. It's what your body uses to build and repair muscles, make enzymes, and even create hormones like estrogen and progesterone.

Try to have a good source of protein with every meal. This doesn't have to be complicated or became a "protein mania." Think eggs with sautéed greens for breakfast, a grilled chicken salad or chickpea bowl for lunch, and maybe a lentil or beans for dinner. On busy days, keep protein-rich snacks like hard-boiled eggs, roasted nuts, or Greek yogurt close at hand to keep you fueled and satisfied.

Protein also helps you with satiety, which is a big help when cravings hit. It steadies your energy and keeps your metabolism humming along.

Fiber: Feed Your Gut, Support Your Mood

Fiber-rich foods, like colorful veggies, whole grains, fruits, and legumes, do more than just keep your digestion regular. They feed all the good bacteria living in your gut, and your gut bacteria actually help regulate inflammation, mood, and hormone breakdown. Eating things like carrots, broccoli, berries, oats, and quinoa supports far more than just filling your tummy.

Including plenty of fiber keeps your blood sugar steady, which helps with mood swings and those sneaky cravings. Try to aim for a variety of colors on your plate, because each color brings different nutrients and plant compounds that support your body in different ways.

Healthy Fats: The Quiet Powerhouses

Not all fats are created equal, and healthy fats are important allies in this journey. Foods high in omega-3s, such as think salmon, walnuts, or flax seeds, as well as monounsaturated fats from olive oil and avocados, help reduce inflammation and keep your cells flexible.

Including healthy fats daily can also support your skin, your mood, and even your nervous system. Don't be afraid to add that drizzle of olive oil to your salad or enjoy some nut butter on your toast.

Flexible and Intuitive Eating: Trusting Your Body Again

You may find that rigid diet plans or obsessively counting calories only add stress during perimenopause, and stress is precisely what you want to avoid. Instead, try checking in with your body's hunger and fullness signals. Ask yourself questions like: Am I really hungry? Am I eating because I'm bored, stressed, or tired?

Giving yourself permission to enjoy the foods you crave, without guilt or worry, helps you rebuild a trusting relationship with food. Mindful eating can help slow down, savor flavors and textures, and really notice how food makes you feel in your body and in your mood.

Mindful eating is all about learning the dance between your body's needs and your mind's messages.

Meal Anchors: Make Eating Easy and Reliable

When your schedule is tight and your energy feels low, making decisions about food can become overwhelming. That's where "meal anchors" come in. These are simple, familiar meals or bowls you like, know how to put together, and can rely on without second-guessing.

Batch cooking or prepping ingredients on weekends can save you time and mental energy during the week. Roast a big tray of veggies, cook a pot of lentils or quinoa, and slice up fresh salad greens. These are all ingredients you can mix and match. Also, keep pantry staples like canned beans, frozen greens, or nuts handy.

Here are some easy meal anchors you can rotate:

- Crambled eggs with spinach

- Greek yogurt topped with fruits and nuts

When eating feels simple and nourishing, it becomes easier to stay consistent without adding more stress.

Nourishing Foods for Hormonal Health in Perimenopause

What you eat plays a huge role in how your body feels and functions during perimenopause. Hormonal shifts can affect how your metabolism works, your energy levels, mood, and even your cravings. Choosing the right foods helps support your body through these changes. It can help to stabilize blood sugar, reduce inflammation, support hormone production, and nurture your gut health, which is closely tied to your hormones and mood.

Here's a list of foods that can help you nurture hormonal harmony, along with why they're especially beneficial during perimenopause.

Protein Sources for Balance:

Protein is essential because it provides the amino acids your body needs to produce hormones like estrogen and progesterone. It also helps maintain muscle mass, which tends to decline with hormonal changes, and keeps you feeling full, helping to manage cravings.

- **Eggs:** rich in high-quality protein and healthy fats that support hormone synthesis

- **Chicken and turkey:** lean meats provide essential protein with less saturated fat

- **Fatty fish (salmon, mackerel, and sardines):** full of omega-3 fatty acids that reduce inflammation and support brain and heart health

- **Plant-based proteins (lentils, chickpeas, and black beans):** high in protein and fiber, they help balance blood sugar and provide steady energy

- **Tofu and tempeh:** soy-based proteins contain phytoestrogens that may gently support estrogen balance

- **Greek yogurt and cottage cheese:** dairy sources with protein and probiotics for gut and immune health

- **Nuts and seeds (almonds, walnuts, chia, and flaxseeds):** provide protein, healthy fats, and fiber, feeding your body steadily and supporting hormone production

Fiber-Rich Vegetables and Fruits for a healthy Gut and Stable Mood:

Fiber supports digestion and feeds beneficial gut bacteria, which play a key role in managing inflammation and hormone metabolism. A healthy gut helps regulate your mood and cravings, giving you more control over your appetite.

- **Leafy greens (spinach, kale, and Swiss chard):** packed with vitamins, minerals, and fiber that nourish your body and gut

- **Broccoli, Brussels sprouts, and cauliflower:** cruciferous vegetables found to help with estrogen metabolism, promoting hormonal balance

- **Carrots, sweet potatoes, and butternut squash:** colorful veggies full of antioxidants and fiber to reduce inflammation

- **Berries (blueberries, strawberries, and raspberries):** rich in antioxidants that protect against hormone-related oxidative stress

- **Apples and pears (with skin):** contain fiber and vitamins that help maintain stable blood sugar

- **Avocados:** loaded with fiber and healthy fats that support hormone production and reduce inflammation

Healthy Fats to Help Your Hormones and Boost Your Brain:

Healthy fats are crucial because hormones are made from cholesterol, and fat supports brain function, skin health, while reducing inflammation, all important during perimenopause.

- **Olive oil:** rich in monounsaturated fats and antioxidants that support heart and hormone health

- **Avocado oil:** another source of good fats that reduce inflammation

- **Nuts (almonds, walnuts, and pistachios):** provide essential fatty acids and vitamins supporting hormone production and balanced blood sugar

- **Seeds (flaxseeds, chia seeds, and pumpkin seeds):** contain omega-3s and phytoestrogens that gently support hormone balance

- **Fatty fish (listed above):** supports brain and nervous system health

- **Coconut oil:** contains medium-chain triglycerides that provide quick energy and may support metabolism

Whole Grains for Steady Energy:

Whole grains provide fiber and nutrients that help keep your blood sugar balanced and support digestive health, reducing mood swings and energy crashes.

- **Oats:** slow-digesting carbs that provide steady energy and soothe digestion

- **Quinoa:** a complete protein and rich in fiber and minerals

- **Brown rice, barley, buckwheat, and millet:** all offer fiber and slow-release energy to support balanced metabolism

Other Beneficial Foods to Support Your Whole System:

- **Fermented foods (kimchi, sauerkraut, kefir, and miso):** probiotics promote a healthy gut microbiome, essential for hormone metabolism and emotional health

- **Green tea:** contains antioxidants and modest caffeine that support metabolism without overstimulation

- **Herbs like turmeric and ginger:** natural anti-inflammatories that can ease aches and support hormone health

- **Herbal teas (chamomile and peppermint):** calming and supportive for stress and digestion

- **Water:** staying hydrated helps all of your body systems work efficiently, including hormone transport and detoxification

Foods to Limit or Avoid:

To help your hormones work smoothly, take a break from

- processed and ultra-processed foods.

- excessive caffeine that can disrupt sleep and increase anxiety.

- added sugars and refined carbs.

- excess alcohol, which can interfere with hormone metabolism and sleep quality.

- artificial additives and preservatives that may burden the liver and your overall health.

Remember that eating well during perimenopause is about balance, ease, and showing up for yourself meal by meal, nourishing your body and mind with what it really needs.

Pillar Two: Movement (for Purpose and Vitality)

Movement isn't about punishment or pushing beyond your limits, especially during perimenopause. Instead, it's about honoring what your body needs now: building strength where it's needed, keeping circulation flowing, and calming your nervous system so you feel grounded and energized. The right kind of movement can truly be a game-changer.

As estrogen declines, several things happen inside your body. Your muscle mass naturally decreases, bone density can weaken, metabolism slows down, and mood fluctuations become common. Regular, gentle movement can help to counter these effects. It keeps your muscles strong, bones supported, and mental fog at bay.

Movement doesn't have to mean spending hours at the gym or running marathons. There are many simple, consistent actions you can take to honor your body's changing rhythms and your busy schedule.

Strength Training: The Minimum Effective Dose

You don't have to lift heavy weights or spend hours working out. Research shows that just 15 to 20-minute sessions daily targeting major muscle groups, such as the legs, back, chest, and core, can help preserve muscle and bone health.

As you age and hormones shift, maintaining lean muscle supports a healthy metabolism and steadier energy levels. Strength training also boosts confidence, balance, and overall resilience.

Examples of simple but effective exercises:

- **Bodyweight squats:** Stand with your feet shoulder-width apart, bend your knees and hips to sit back like you're lowering into a chair, keeping your chest lifted. Rise back up. Aim for 10–12 slow, controlled reps.

- **Wall or countertop push-ups:** Face a wall or sturdy countertop, place your hands shoulder-width apart, and lower your chest toward the surface, then push back. Do 8–10 reps.

- **Bent-over rows with light weights or water bottles:** Holding light weights or bottles, hinge forward slightly at the hips, pull your elbows back, squeezing your shoulder blades, then lower. Try to do 10–12 reps at a time.

- **Plank holds:** Lie face down on the floor, then lift yourself onto your forearms or hands, keeping your body straight from head to heels. Start with 20 seconds and gradually build up.

Choose weights or resistance that challenge but don't exhaust you. The last few reps should feel like effort without causing strain or pain.

Walking: The Simple, Secret Reset

Walking is one of the easiest and most beneficial exercises you can do. It's low-impact, fits into any schedule, and offers natural mood-boosting benefits, especially when you step outside.

Walking helps to get your blood flowing, ease joint stiffness, support heart and lung health, and encourage vitamin D production in sunlight. It also calms your nervous system, helping with stress and better sleep later on.

Try to aim for a few short walks daily of between 10 to 15 minutes each, or a longer stroll when you can. Walk during breaks, after meals, or even during phone calls. Focus on keeping a pace where you can still chat comfortably.

Walking should feel like a pleasure, not a chore. Wear comfortable shoes, notice the sights and sounds around you, and let your mind unwind.

Mobility and Breath Breaks to Stay Loose and Calm

Sitting for long hours or being tense from stress can create stiffness and tightness that discourage movement. Brief mobility and breath breaks can reset your body and mind, loosening tight muscles and calming stress hormones.

Try these simple moves right at your desk or in any small space:

- **Shoulder rolls:** Lift your shoulders toward your ears, then roll them back and down slowly 10 times. Reverse direction for 10 more.

- **Neck stretches:** Gently tilt your head toward one shoulder and hold for 15 seconds. Switch sides. Repeat about three times.

- **Hip openers:** While sitting, cross your ankle over your opposite knee and lean forward slightly to stretch your hips. Hold for 20 seconds, then switch your legs.

- **Deep belly breathing:** Place one hand on your belly and one on your chest. Inhale slowly through your nose, feel your belly rise, then exhale gently through pursed lips, watching the belly fall. Repeat five times.

Breath-focused resets work wonders for calming the nervous system and clearing mental fog. Use them during moments of overwhelm or before challenging tasks.

Simple Movement Ideas for Busy Days

Life can get hectic, especially when you're juggling work, family, and self-care. But even busy days can have pockets of movement:

- Use TV commercial breaks to stand and do stretches or light strength moves like squats or wall push-ups.

- Walk in place or march gently during phone calls or meetings.

- Use waiting times in lines or traffic to practice slow, mindful breathing or gentle stretches.

- Take a short mid-afternoon walk outside for a mental reset.

The key is to move whenever you can, even if it's just five minutes at a time. Little bursts of activity add up.

Listening to Your Body: Movement for Today

Some days your energy will be high, and you'll feel ready for a brisk walk or strength session. Other days, your body might need gentle stretches or mindful breathing. Both high-engagement and restorative movement are valuable. The goal is to stay connected, honor your limits, and build consistency over time.

Movement is your tool for vitality, not punishment. Finding joy and ease in moving your body will encourage you to keep it up, supporting your hormones, your mood, and your whole self.

Pillar Three: Stress (Managing the Invisible Load)

Stress can be sneaky. It doesn't always announce itself with a big, dramatic event. Instead, it creeps into your day through countless small moments, such as racing thoughts, endless to-do lists, social pressures, multitasking, and digital overwhelm. During perimenopause, your body and mind are already dealing with so much change that stress can easily tip the balance, affecting your hormones, mood, sleep, and even how you eat.

If this invisible load isn't managed, it can undo all the good work you're doing with eating, moving, and sleeping. But the great news is that stress can also be managed, often in just a few minutes here and there, and those small moments of care add up to big improvements.

Recognize Hidden Stress

Stress isn't just the big life stuff like deadlines or conflicts. It's also the background noise in your head telling you're not doing enough or that things are overwhelming. Maybe it's the mental chatter you don't even notice anymore, or the pressure you feel scrolling through social media comparing yourself to others. Sometimes it's just being pulled in too many directions at once.

The first step is noticing when you're tense. Are your shoulders tight? Is your breathing shallow? Does your mind feel like it's spinning? Recognizing these signs early lets you step in with kindness instead of letting stress build until it crashes your mood or energy.

Micro-Practices With Big Impact

You don't need a yoga retreat or hours of meditation to reduce stress. Small moments of mindfulness and breath can reset your system anywhere, whether you're at your desk, your kitchen, or even in the car.

- **Diaphragmatic breathing:** Take two minutes to breathe slowly and deeply into your belly. Place one hand on your belly and one on your chest. Inhale deeply through your nose, feeling your belly rise like a balloon filling with air. Exhale slowly through pursed lips, letting your belly fall. Repeat this for a couple of minutes. This simple act calms your brain and body, lowering your cortisol levels.

- **Mindful micro-breaks:** Noticing your senses brings you back to the present moment, out of stress loops and into calm. For example, pause and list:

    - five things you can see

    - four things you can touch

    - three sounds you hear

    - two smells in the air

- one taste or sensation in your mouth

This simple exercise grounds your mind in the present, easing tension and clearing mental fog.

Interrupt Automatic Stress Patterns

Stress often triggers automatic reactions, often a sharp word, a snack binge, or rushing through tasks. While these responses may bring instant relief, they can actually make things worse. You can stop this cycle by becoming curious before acting.

Start identifying your common stress triggers: maybe it's an unexpected email, a critical comment, or watching the clock tick down on a deadline. When you notice the trigger, pause. Take a breath, and ask yourself questions like: What's actually happening? What's the best way to respond?

Sometimes just stepping away for a minute for a short walk, a sip of water, or a deep breath helps reframe your perspective and calm your nervous system. This practice rewires your brain over time, helping you respond with clarity rather than react.

Build Resilience Gradually

Managing stress is a skill that grows with practice. You build reserves that help you bounce back faster from life's ups and downs.

Start with small habits: Journal your feelings a few minutes a day to get them out of your head and into perspective. Practice gratitude by noting one thing you're thankful for each morning or evening. Set boundaries kindly and say "no" when your plate's full, or ask for help when you need it.

These simple acts can make you less emotionally reactive and strengthen your nervous system. Over time, stress will feel more manageable, moods will stabilize, and your energy will improve.

Pillar Four: Sleep (The Essential Reset)

Sleep is your body's nightly reset button. When you get a good night's rest, your brain clears out the clutter, your hormones that control hunger and fullness (leptin and ghrelin) find balance, your mood steadies, and your body gets to work repairing cells and tissues. But as hormones change during perimenopause, sleep often feels like one of the first things to go. Night sweats, racing thoughts, or just an inability to fall or stay asleep can leave you feeling exhausted and foggy the next day.

The good news is that even small improvements in how you prepare for bed and your sleep environment can have a big impact on how rested you feel. It's less about getting "perfect" sleep and more about creating a calming, consistent routine that supports your natural rhythms.

Prioritize a Wind-Down Routine

Screens and sleep don't mix. The blue light from phones, tablets, and laptops tricks your brain into thinking it's still daytime, blocking the release of melatonin, the hormone that tells your body that it's time to rest. Aim to switch off screens 30 to 60 minutes before bed.

During this time, dim the lights and do something relaxing like sipping chamomile or lavender tea. Gentle stretches or reading a favorite book (paper pages, not backlit screens) are great ways to signal to your body that the day is winding down.

Try creating a little ritual each night, for example, lighting a candle, journaling a few gratitude notes, or listening to soft music. These cues train your brain to associate the routine with rest.

Regularity Is Key

Your body loves predictability. Going to bed and waking up at the same time, even on weekends, helps keep your internal clock steady.

Skipping around with sleep times confuses your circadian rhythm and can leave you feeling groggy and out of sync.

Try setting a bedtime that feels right for you and a wake time you can stick to during the week. That might mean leaving technology out of your bed or setting an alarm to remind you to start your wind-down ritual.

Optimize Your Sleep Environment

The bedroom should be a sanctuary for rest. Make it cool, dark, and quiet. Use blackout curtains to block streetlights, a white noise machine or a fan if ambient noise bugs you, and comfortable bedding that suits your preferences.

Save your bed for sleep and intimacy only. You shouldn't be working, scrolling on your phone, or watching TV there. This helps your brain build a strong link between bed and resting.

Calm the Mind

Sleep struggles often come with a busy, anxious mind. If you find yourself lying awake with racing thoughts, try progressive muscle relaxation. This means tensing one muscle group at a time, holding briefly, then releasing slowly, from your toes all the way up to your face.

Alternatively, guided meditation apps can lead you gently into relaxation. Simple focused breathing with slow, deep inhales and exhales can also slow your heart rate and quiet your mind.

It's okay if these techniques don't knock you out right away. Like exercise, sleep habits take time and practice. The goal is for you to create a calm transition from wakefulness to rest.

Small Wins, Big Impact

You don't have to overhaul your sleep overnight. Even adding 15 minutes of good sleep, or reducing how often you wake up, can make you feel brighter and your energy levels steadier in the mornings.

Notice what shifts feel the most doable. Maybe it's a 10-minute pre-bed ritual, drawing curtains earlier, or turning off your phone at 9 p.m. Celebrate those wins because every gentle step helps build your body's ability to rest and heal.

Pillar Five: Emotions (and relationships)

Perimenopause can turn up the volume on your emotions like a dial you can't quite control. Some days, small irritations feel overwhelming, while at other moments, joy or sadness come rushing in without warning. Hormonal shifts affect brain chemicals that regulate mood, so your feelings can feel bigger and more unpredictable.

The key isn't trying to push those feelings away or to judge yourself for being "too emotional." Instead, it's about learning how to work with your emotions with kindness and awareness. By tuning into your feelings and gently responding rather than reacting, you build emotional resilience that flows through all aspects of your life.

Pause and Name Your Feelings

You don't need to carve out extra time to practice emotional awareness. You can use simple moments during your day to pause and check in with yourself. Maybe it's brushing your teeth, waiting for your coffee to brew, or standing in line at the store.

Ask yourself: What am I feeling right now? It might be irritation, joy, anxiety, or peacefulness. The goal isn't to judge the emotion or change it, but just to name it. Recognizing your feelings is the first step toward understanding and managing them.

Over time, this habit helps you spot emotional patterns, such as times of day, situations, or people that tend to bring up certain feelings. This helps you better prepare for and care for yourself.

Journal to Track Patterns

Keeping a brief journal can deepen your emotional insight. Jot down what triggered a strong feeling and how you responded. Did taking a deep breath help calm you? Did you lash out and then regret it? Did you reach out to a friend, or did you need to retreat for some quiet time?

Reflecting on what helps or hinders your emotional balance builds your emotional toolbox. You start noticing what supports your well-being and what adds fuel to the fire.

Shift Your Inner Voice

It's easy for self-talk to turn harsh, especially during tough days. When you catch yourself thinking things like, *I'm failing*, or *I'm too emotional*, try gently shifting those thoughts:

- Replace "I'm failing" with "I'm doing the best I can with what I have right now."
- Instead of "I'm too emotional", say "My feelings are messages that tell me what I need."

This reframing creates space for kindness and realism. Your emotions are signals from your body and mind asking for care, rest, or a change.

Be Your Own Best Friend

Imagine how you'd talk to a dear friend who is struggling emotionally. You'd likely offer warmth, understanding, and encouragement, not criticism or blame. That same kindness is exactly what you need to give yourself.

Self-compassion lowers your stress hormones, reduces shame, and builds resilience. When you stumble or feel overwhelmed, instead of spiraling into "I shouldn't be feeling this," soften your inner voice: "This is hard, and that's okay. I'm doing my best."

Practices like reminding yourself of your shared humanity ("Many women have these feelings"), gentle self-talk, and small acts of kindness, like a warm bath or quiet time, help nurture your emotional health in powerful ways.

Mastering emotional self-leadership is a journey. It doesn't mean you won't have intense feelings or bad days. It means learning to meet those emotions with curiosity and care, guiding yourself back to balance softly and steadily.

Pillar Six: Imbalances (Habits That no Longer Serve your Body)

This pillar focuses on everyday habits and behaviors that quietly chip away at your well-being. Think of these as the little things that pile up, such as a bit too much caffeine, late-night scrolling on your phone, mindless snacking on processed foods, chaotic schedules, working too hard without rest, or those reward loops where you reach for a treat to cope with stress.

These behavioral excesses ripple through your life, messing up your sleep, stirring up cravings, wobbling your moods, and weakening your ability to regulate your emotions and energy. They can amplify symptoms you're already experiencing during perimenopause, making things feel heavier and more overwhelming than they need to be.

Listen Closely to Your Body's Signals

Your body is constantly sending messages. If you're tired all the time, snappy with loved ones, craving sugar at strange hours, or can't seem to settle down for sleep, these are red flags. Imbalance often shows up before a full-blown crisis. Learning to notice these early signals helps you catch problems when they're easier to handle.

Do you find yourself reaching for that second (or third) cup of coffee to get through the afternoon slump? Or staying up late scrolling through social media, only to regret it when you wake up foggy. Perhaps you're constantly battling overwhelm because your calendar feels chaotic. These aren't just annoyances. They add up and affect your entire system.

Track and Reflect to Create Awareness

One of the most powerful steps you can take is becoming aware of the habits that might be contributing to your imbalance. Keep a simple log, either on a note on your phone or a small notebook, where you jot down moments you feel drained, irritable, or craving unhealthy foods. Also, make a note of what you were doing, for example, "Had a triple espresso at 3 p.m.," "Stayed on phone until midnight," or "Skipped lunch, then binged on snacks."

This practice helps you spot patterns that might otherwise feel invisible. Once habits are in sight, they lose some of their power, and you gain the freedom to make different choices.

Small, Gentle Corrections Cascade Through Your Health

Changing these habits doesn't mean drastic deprivation or harsh rules. The goal is to apply small, realistic tweaks that add up over time and restore balance across all the other pillars.

Maybe this means swapping your usual mid-afternoon coffee for a calming herbal tea a few days a week. Or setting a gentle "tech curfew" by putting your devices away 30 minutes before bed to improve sleep quality. Perhaps it's scheduling a 10-minute walk after meals that becomes your new go-to for clearing mental fog.

These small choices can create ripple effects. Better sleep means calmer moods, fewer cravings, and more energy to move or relax. Reducing screen time can lower stress and improve your emotional regulation. With tiny, manageable shifts, you start restoring harmony and taking back control.

Respect Your Limits

One of the toughest lessons can be recognizing that rest is how you maintain everything else. When your days feel overloaded, saying "no" becomes an act of self-care, not failure. Delegating tasks, setting boundaries at work or home, and protecting downtime are vital ways to sustain your health.

Remind yourself that rest fuels productivity, mood, and overall well-being. It's okay to slow down. Listening to your body and honoring your limits helps avoid burnout and keeps all the pillars strong.

Perimenopause invites you to notice the habits that no longer serve your evolving body and mind. By identifying these imbalances and gently correcting course, you restore stability not just in this pillar, but across your whole life, helping you feel more grounded, balanced, and ready to thrive.

Bringing It All Together: Synergy and Sustainable Change

The six pillars are like threads woven together to create a strong safety net for your health. When you improve one area, it often helps lift others as well. For example, getting better sleep can stabilize your mood and reduce cravings. Moving your body regularly helps you sleep more deeply. Managing stress makes it easier to focus and stay emotionally balanced. Cutting back on habits that throw you off frees up energy to eat well, move, and rest.

Remember, this is about making small, caring choices that add up over time. Each thoughtful step you take, day by day, builds strength and helps you move more smoothly through perimenopause and beyond.

Building Your Balanced Reset

Starting a reset during perimenopause helps you to build a balanced lifestyle that supports you every day. Think of it as creating a firm foundation made up of small, consistent habits that honor your body's shifting needs and your busy schedule.

These exercises will help you take everything you've learned about the six pillars and turn it into practical, doable steps. It's about finding balance, not perfection, and making a reset that fits your life, your priorities, and the unique rhythm you're living right now.

Six Pillars Self-Assessment

Rate your current status on each pillar from 1 (needs attention) to 5 (strong), then write one small action you can take for each pillar to support balance this week.

Pillar	**Current rating (1-5)**	**Small next step**
Eating		
Movement		
Stress		
Sleep		
Emotions		
Imbalances		

Identify and Interrupt Imbalance Loops

List habits or patterns that tend to throw off your balance, for example, late-night scrolling or emotional eating. For each, write:

What triggers it?

____

How does it impact the other pillars?

What one small, actionable step can I take to interrupt or replace the habit?

Build a Mini Daily Routine Incorporating the Six Pillars

Design a simple daily routine with at least one small action from each pillar that feels doable for your current energy and schedule. Include specific times or anchors, for example:

- morning protein-rich breakfast (eating)
- 10 minutes of stretching or walking (movement)
- mid-morning breathing pause (stress)
- consistent 10 p.m. bedtime (sleep)
- journaling a mood check-in (emotions)

- turning off screens by 9:30 p.m. (imbalances)

Building your balanced reset is a journey, not a finish line. Celebrate each small habit you add and every moment you listen to yourself with kindness. Over time, these steady steps add up to big changes: more energy, better mood, deeper rest, and greater ease through perimenopause and beyond. Keep returning to your pillars, adjust as you go, and remember that this reset isn't just about surviving this phase, but thriving in it.

Final Thoughts

Now that you understand how the six lifestyle pillars work together to support you during perimenopause, you can begin to include these practical, time-efficient strategies into your daily routine. Embracing small, compassionate changes in each area helps create a steady foundation that honors your body's shifting needs without adding pressure or complexity.

By tuning in to your real hunger, moving with intention, managing stress in bite-sized moments, prioritizing restful sleep, guiding your emotional waves with kindness, and gently correcting habits that throw you off balance, you set yourself up for greater energy, resilience, and ease. This helps to build a flexible framework that grows stronger with every mindful step, preparing you for a smoother transition through perimenopause and beyond.

Chapter 5:

Emotional Eating as Regulation—Decode Triggers and Begin Gentle Rewiring

Have you ever found yourself reaching for a snack without really feeling hungry, then wondered what triggered that urge? Maybe it's a wave of stress after a long workday or the quiet moments when the house feels too empty. Or perhaps you notice patterns, such as a certain time of day, a particular mood, or an event, that seem to nudge you toward eating even when your body doesn't need fuel. These are the subtle signals of emotional hunger, often tangled up with our feelings and daily rhythms in ways that can feel confusing and automatic.

What if you could start to recognize these triggers, understand what's really behind those cravings, and gently shift your habits without judgment or pressure? Let's explore those hidden patterns with kindness and curiosity, offering new tools to listen to your body and emotions more clearly. It's about learning how to pause, notice, experiment, and build trust in yourself as you navigate the unique changes perimenopause brings.

Biological vs. Emotional Hunger

One of the biggest challenges during perimenopause is learning to tell the difference between biological hunger, your body's real need for fuel, and emotional hunger, which is tied to feelings rather than physical need. Knowing the difference helps you respond in ways that truly support your well-being.

What Is Biological Hunger?

Biological hunger is your body's natural signal telling you it needs energy. It usually builds gradually and feels physical:

- a quiet emptiness or growling in your stomach
- a sense of lightheadedness or difficulty concentrating
- sometimes a low mood or irritability linked to low blood sugar
- relief and satisfaction when you eat enough nutritious food

Biological hunger grows steadily and can be satisfied by almost any healthy, nourishing food. It urges you to eat for energy and repair, helping you stay strong during hormonal changes.

What Is Emotional Hunger?

Emotional hunger comes from feelings, not physical need. It often happens suddenly and can feel urgent:

- cravings for specific comfort foods, like sweets or salty snacks
- eating triggered by stress, boredom, loneliness, or fatigue
- eating even when your stomach feels full or comfortable
- feeling a temporary relief or distraction after eating, followed by guilt or emptiness

Emotional hunger seeks something that gives emotional comfort or soothes uneasy feelings. It often comes on quickly and can be linked to specific situations or moods.

How to Spot the Differences

Here are some ways to tell biological and emotional hunger apart:

Biological hunger	**Emotional hunger**
comes on gradually	comes on suddenly
can wait a bit before eating	feels urgent, hard to ignore
physical cues like stomach growling	triggered by emotions or situations
open to a variety of foods	craves specific foods
eating satisfies and ends hunger	eating may not satisfy or lead to guilt

Learning to differentiate these hungers is a key part of building a healthier, more compassionate relationship with food during perimenopause. With practice, you can honor your body's true needs and gently care for your emotional well-being.

Mapping Emotional Eating Patterns and Triggers

Constantly wanting to have a snack, grabbing unhealthy food choices, and feeling hungry shortly after eating are some of the most common challenges women in perimenopause struggle with.

Most emotional eating happens through automatic patterns running quietly in the background of your day. You might feel like a passenger in your own eating habits, confused about what triggers the urge, or frustrated because it feels out of your control. But emotional eating doesn't have to be a mystery.

By bringing gentle, curious attention to these patterns, you can start to see them clearly. Instead of tracking food to restrict or judge yourself, think of tracking as a compassionate act of self-discovery. Writing down your experiences without blame or criticism turns eating from a source of frustration into a window for understanding and kindness. You begin to shift the story from self-blame to genuine insight.

Emotional eating usually starts with a trigger that leads you to seek comfort in food. These triggers aren't always dramatic events. They often arise from everyday moments, such as the post-lunch slump during a long workday, the quiet after the household settles down, or a tense conversation with a partner.

For example, you might notice that a snack becomes irresistible after a marathon of Zoom meetings, or that a bowl of ice cream feels like the only way to fill the silence once the kids are in bed or the house is finally quiet. Sometimes, emotional eating hides behind feelings of invisibility or unacknowledged effort. When no one seems to notice your hard work, food quietly steps in as a source of comfort. It's not always negative: food can be a way to celebrate, reward, or soothe after a taxing week.

Think about your life and what might trigger your emotional eating. Naming these moments helps you step back and create space between what you're feeling and how you're responding. Recognizing patterns, like realizing you always crave snacks while watching TV alone or reach for comfort food during stressful work calls, gives you the power to change what comes next.

A food-emotion diary is a kind, non-judgmental tool to support this discovery. Simple daily notes can include:

- time of eating
- whether the hunger is physical or emotional
- what emotion or situation was present

- what food was eaten

Here is an example diary entry:

- **Time:** 9:00 p.m.
- **Hunger:** 2 (0-10)
- **Emotion or situation:** feeling lonely while scrolling social media in a quiet house
- **Food:** one bowl of ice cream

Writing these details without trying to explain or fix anything opens doors to understanding. After just a few days, you may spot repeating loops: the evening when the quiet of the evening triggers sweet cravings or the mid-afternoon snack after a work marathon.

These habits form because your brain learns that certain behaviors bring comfort during stress, making those pathways automatic. What starts as a rare treat can become a go-to response, but awareness is the first step to gentle change.

Once you see the pattern, you can ask: "What else might bring comfort or manage stress in this moment?" This approach encourages you to think about your life and what you want, and invites experimentation rather than harsh self-control.

Even a few days of tracking can shift your relationship with food from frustration to kindness. Each entry builds self-compassion, opening the way for small, sustainable changes that honor where you are right now.

Mindful, Intuitive Eating as a Foundation

Eating well during perimenopause is about giving yourself the tools to listen to your body and respond with kindness. These principles create space for gentler, thoughtful eating that honors your changing needs.

Pause and Notice Before You Eat

Before brushing off hunger as just a habit or giving in to cravings automatically, take a moment to check in with yourself.

- Ask yourself: "Am I physically hungry, or am I eating because I feel bored, stressed, or tired?"

- During your meal, pause occasionally and rate your fullness on a scale from 1 to 10.

- After eating, notice how your body feels. Are you satisfied or still hungry?

- This simple pause helps you rebuild trust in your body's natural signals, which hormones often confuse during perimenopause.

Taking moments to pause and check in with your hunger and fullness is a simple but powerful way to reconnect with your body's needs. These pauses build trust and help you make choices that support nourishment and balance.

Removing Moral Language Around Food

Calling foods "good," "bad," "healthy" or "junk" adds guilt to eating and sets up harmful cycles of restriction and binging. This only makes emotional eating worse, especially during hormonal shifts. Here are a few strategies you can incorporate:

- Shift your mindset. Food is neutral. It provides energy, comfort, and pleasure. None of these deserves judgment.

- Instead of "I shouldn't have eaten that," try "I noticed I wanted something sweet, so I chose a piece of chocolate. Did it satisfy me?"

- Replace rigid rules like "I must eat clean" with questions like "What would feel nourishing and satisfying right now?"

Over time, your inner voice becomes a curious, kind friend rather than a harsh critic, inviting gentle choices.

Letting go of "good" and "bad" labels around food frees you from guilt and opens up space for kindness. Embracing food as neutral empowers you to make peaceful, less stressful choices that honor your body and mind.

Emphasizing Pleasure and Satisfaction

Eating is about more than nourishment. It's also about joy, comfort, and feeling grounded. When you ignore pleasure, your body often craves more intense flavors or bigger portions. Here are a few tips to bring enjoyment to your meals:

- Slow down and savor each bite, paying attention to taste, texture, and aroma.
- Notice when your enjoyment peaks. That's often the sign to stop.
- Allow yourself small pleasures, like a square of dark chocolate or a creamy dressing, to avoid feeling deprived later and chasing more food.
- Eating without distraction, even just a few bites, helps you tune in to satisfaction and reduce overeating.

Including pleasure in your meals is essential. When you savor your food, you're more likely to feel satisfied and less likely to reach for extra snacks. Pleasure and nourishment go hand in hand.

Building Meal Anchors

Perimenopause can throw off your appetite and your eating schedules, but having loosely structured meal anchors provides stability.

- Aim for regular meals built around:

    - protein (eggs, beans, chicken, or tofu)
    - fiber (whole grains, vegetables, or fruit)
    - color (leafy greens, peppers, or berries)
- Examples include:
    - **Breakfast:** scrambled eggs with spinach and whole wheat toast
    - **Lunch:** grilled chicken, brown rice, and roasted vegetables
    - **Dinner:** quinoa bowl with chickpeas, tomatoes, cucumber, and lemon-tahini dressing
- For snacks, try Greek yogurt with berries or nuts and fruit.
- A gentle eating rhythm prevents skipping meals and helps steady mood and energy.

Creating regular, balanced meal anchors gives your day structure and steadiness, easing blood sugar swings and mood dips. These simple habits help you navigate perimenopause with more ease and confidence.

As you practice these principles, eating shifts from feeling like a battle to becoming a mindful, caring moment. This foundation supports you in making small, compassionate changes guided by curiosity and self-trust. Each meal is a step toward deeper understanding and a more peaceful relationship with food.

Behavior Change Experiments, Self-Compassion, and Tracking Tools

The foundation of mindful and intuitive eating builds the base for every experiment in this chapter. These changes work not because they demand strict rules, but because they invite curiosity and allow room for your own wisdom. Feeling an urge to eat when emotions are high is normal, and interrupting that reflex with compassion changes the pattern over time.

The Power of Pause Experiment

When you sense the urge to eat, give yourself permission to pause for a short while. Imagine you're standing in the pantry after a tough work call, maybe your muscles are tense, and your thoughts are swirling. At this moment, place your hand over your chest or belly. Take 5 or 10 slow, deep breaths. Feel your feet pressing into the floor. Notice what is happening in your body, for example, tight shoulders, a quickening heart, and maybe a lump in your throat. This creates just enough space for choice. You might realize the craving softens as you breathe, or you might decide you truly are hungry and reach for something comforting with awareness.

Here are the steps you can take:

1. When an urge hits, stop before you act.
2. Stand or sit still, and place your hand on your body where you feel the sensation of the urge.
3. Take slow, deep breaths, counting each inhale and exhale up to 10. Notice your body and mind without judgment.

This simple pause creates a powerful space between urge and action. With practice, it strengthens your ability to listen deeply to your body and mind, helping you respond with awareness rather than rushing into old habits. Each breath is a step toward greater self-kindness and choice.

Curiosity Over Control

Self-compassion starts with curiosity. Instead of judging yourself for emotional eating, try observing your experience like a caring guide. Maybe you've noticed yourself reaching for cookies at night. Pause for a moment and ask: What am I really needing right now? Is it rest, comfort, or a simple pause from the day? By noticing without blame, you begin to respond with care instead of guilt.

Observation alone can be powerful. You might discover that your strongest cravings come late at night, when you feel tired or alone. Simply acknowledging this pattern opens up new options, such as calling a friend, reading a few pages of a book, or sitting quietly with a warm cup of tea.

Rigid rules around food often make things harder. Perimenopause brings changes in energy, moods, and appetite. Letting yourself enjoy dessert, or another small pleasure, is a way of trusting your body and your instincts. Over time, the sense of restriction eases, and the power of "forbidden" foods naturally fades.

Supportive Self-Talk Practice

Build a habit of kind language. Affirmations and gentle reminders lift your spirit and soften the edge of hard moments. Phrases like "I am learning to listen to my body" or "Every pause matters" can ease shame and encourage patience. Return to these words during struggles, as they make space for kindness and encourage resilience.

Behavioral Pattern Map and Food-Emotion Diary

Map your patterns with a journal designed for gentle, ongoing practice rather than keeping score.

Include things like:

Time of day:

___

Emotion before eating:

___

___

Physical sensations or hunger cues:

____

____

____

____

Food chosen:

____

____

____

____

Notes on what happened, what I discovered, and ideas for next time.

____

____

____

____

Reflect daily or weekly:

What emotions tend to spark eating?

____

____

____

____

Which alternatives felt nurturing?

____

____

____

____

____

How did the urge feel before and after a gentle pause or substitute actions?

____

____

____

____

____

This process isn't about perfection. Every day brings new chances to learn and grow, with tracking as your companion for self-trust and gradual, meaningful change.

Final Thoughts

Now that you've learned to recognize the difference between physical and emotional hunger, mapped your unique triggers, and practiced mindful eating with kindness and curiosity, you're ready to take gentle steps toward lasting change. By treating each urge as an opportunity to pause, explore, and experiment, rather than a moment of failure, you build trust in yourself and your body's signals. Small, compassionate experiments help you discover what truly nourishes and satisfies you, making it easier to break old patterns without harsh judgment or strict rules.

As you continue tracking and reflecting, you'll strengthen your ability to respond to perimenopause's challenges with resilience and self-compassion, creating a foundation for healthier habits and a smoother transition into this new phase of your life.

Chapter 6:

Mental Health First Aid—Stabilizing Mood, Memory, and Focus With Emotional Self-Leadership

Mood swings, memory lapses, and trouble focusing are often seen as signs of weakness or simple aging, but what if they're actually signals from your brain asking for a different kind of care? During perimenopause, these changes are more than just occasional glitches. They're part of a complex shift in how your hormones interact with your brain's chemistry. Recognizing this can turn frustration into understanding and open the door to new ways of managing your mental and emotional life.

Let's explore how hormonal fluctuations affect your mood, memory, and concentration, and use practical, science-based tools to help you navigate the ups and downs with greater ease. You'll discover how developing emotional self-leadership skills, such as mindful awareness, breath control, and setting healthy boundaries, can stabilize your inner world. With approaches specifically adapted to your busy life, you'll learn how to build resilience, sharpen focus, and regain a sense of balance that supports both your mental clarity and emotional well-being during this unique phase.

Understanding Emotional and Cognitive Changes

Perimenopause brings with it a wave of emotional, cognitive, and psychological shifts. You might notice changes in how quickly your emotions shift, experience moments of forgetfulness that seem unusual for you, or have difficulty concentrating on tasks that once felt easy. These experiences can be confusing and might lead to worries that something is wrong with you or that you're losing your mind.

These changes are caused by very real hormonal fluctuations in your body. As your estrogen levels rise and fall irregularly and your progesterone levels gradually decrease, your brain's chemistry gets affected. This, in turn, influences your mood, your ability to remember details, how you manage stress, and even your ability to focus. Your brain and nervous system are adapting to a new hormonal environment, which can temporarily disrupt the way your emotions and thoughts flow.

Understanding that these shifts have biological roots can help to reassure you and reduce the sense of isolation you might feel. This period of transition invites you to approach yourself with compassion and curiosity to create the reset, rather than judgment or fear. With that awareness, you can develop tools and strategies to support your emotional and cognitive health, helping you go through perimenopause with greater clarity and ease.

How Hormonal Shifts Affect Your Emotions

Fluctuating estrogen and progesterone affect your neurotransmitters like serotonin and dopamine, the chemicals in your brain that regulate calmness, motivation, and emotional steadiness. When hormone levels rise and fall unpredictably, your emotional landscape can shift just as quickly.

You may notice:

- sudden irritability
- unexpected sadness

- anxiety that seems to appear out of nowhere
- emotional reactions that feel "too big" for the moment

Recognizing these changes for what they are helps you meet yourself with patience instead of guilt.

Memory, Focus, and the "Foggy Mind" Feeling

As you go through perimenopause, you may experience what's often called "brain fog," a fuzzy, forgetful, or scattered feeling that can affect your daily functioning. This is due to a real change in how your brain processes information.

Estrogen plays an essential role in your brain's health, particularly in the hippocampus and prefrontal cortex. These regions are responsible for memory formation, attention, learning, planning, and problem-solving, essentially your brain's core executive functions. When your estrogen levels fluctuate or decrease, these areas don't communicate quite as effectively, leading to the "brain fog."

You might find yourself forgetting familiar names or struggling to keep your train of thought during conversations. Small but important details can slip through the cracks, such as missing appointments or misplacing your keys more than usual. Reading can become a challenge as you may need to reread paragraphs multiple times to fully grasp the meaning. At times, your mind might feel slowed down or scattered, making multitasking or organizing complex tasks much harder than before.

While these cognitive shifts are usually temporary and improve as your body adjusts to hormonal changes, they can still be intensely frustrating, especially when you're juggling work pressures, family responsibilities, or social engagements. Feeling mentally slowed can chip away at your confidence and leave you questioning whether you're still capable of doing certain things.

Knowing that these experiences are a natural part of perimenopause can help you approach them with patience and implement strategies to support your brain health and sharpen your focus, which we'll explore further in this chapter.

How Sleep Disruptions Impact Mental Well-being

Sleep is important to both your emotional and cognitive health, yet it often becomes difficult to get proper rest during perimenopause. Hormonal fluctuations, especially changes in your estrogen and progesterone, can disrupt your natural sleep patterns in several ways. You might find it increasingly difficult to fall asleep at night, or you may wake up frequently and struggle to fall back asleep. Even when you do manage to sleep, the rest may feel light or unrefreshing, leaving you feeling as though you haven't truly recharged.

Missing out on deep, restorative sleep has a big effect on your brain's ability to function optimally. When you don't sleep properly, your emotional resilience decreases. You can become more irritable, and feelings of anxiety or overwhelm can become harder to manage. At the same time, your cognitive functions, including your concentration, memory, and decision-making, take a significant hit. Tasks that once felt straightforward may seem daunting, and it might be tougher to stay focused or recall important details.

Then there's the relationship between sleep and your mood. Poor sleep worsens emotional symptoms, and unresolved stress or anxiety can make it more difficult for you to fall and stay asleep, creating a challenging loop. Understanding this connection is crucial because it encourages you to practice more self-compassion. Rather than blaming yourself for feeling off or foggy, you can start recognizing tiredness as a contributing factor and perhaps your body signaling that it needs attention.

Even small improvements in sleep quality can lead to noticeable improvements in your mental clarity and emotional balance. Simple habits that we discussed in Chapter 4, such as establishing a consistent bedtime routine, reducing screen time before bed, or creating a calming environment, can help shift this cycle over time.

The Stress–Hormone Feedback Loop

Perimenopause doesn't just bring hormonal changes related to estrogen and progesterone, but it also affects how your body handles stress. Cortisol, often called the "stress hormone," plays a crucial role in how your body reacts to everyday pressures. Normally, cortisol helps prepare you to face challenges by increasing alertness and energy in the short term. However, during perimenopause, your body may have a harder time regulating cortisol levels, creating a loop that causes more stress and makes it more difficult to control your emotions.

What this means for you, day to day, is that challenges may feel heavier or more overwhelming than they used to. Tasks or interactions that once seemed manageable might now feel like major hurdles. With heightened sensitivity, even small stressors, like a tense conversation, a looming deadline, or a minor inconvenience, can cause you to overreact.

This stress–hormone loop can also affect how your brain works. When your cortisol spikes, your memory, focus, and ability to process information can take a hit. You might notice it's harder to concentrate, remember details, or stay on top of tasks. Feeling this way can make you doubt yourself and add to the emotional load you're already carrying.

Recognizing this loop is a powerful step toward managing your stress more effectively. Instead of trying to "push through" on willpower alone, you can start using intentional tools to calm your nervous system. Practices like mindful breathing, progressive muscle relaxation, or reframing your thoughts help regulate your stress response. These strategies give you the chance to respond thoughtfully, rather than react impulsively or feel overwhelmed.

As you practice breaking the cycle, you strengthen your resilience and protect your mental and emotional well-being, helping you navigate perimenopause with greater ease and confidence.

Emotion Regulation Skills for Resilience

Regulating your emotions isn't about suppressing your feelings or not allowing yourself to experience them. Instead, it's about guiding your nervous system so you can respond rather than react. These skills are especially powerful during perimenopause, when emotional intensity can rise unexpectedly.

Each practice below strengthens your emotional stability. Think of it like building a muscle in the gym. With every repetition of a certain exercise, that muscle will get stronger. Similarly, every time you work on managing your emotions, you're increasing your ability to accept difficult feelings and respond calmly, which is a skill you can rely on long after menopause.

Mindful Awareness: Creating Space Between Emotion and Reaction

Mindful awareness helps you notice your feelings without being swept away by them. Simply naming what you feel, for example, “I'm tense,” “I'm anxious,” or “I'm overwhelmed,” reduces your brain's alarm response and increases clarity. Let's look at an easy exercise you can do anywhere:

A Three-Minute Body Scan:

Tuning into your body can help you catch early signs of stress or emotional overwhelm before they take over your day. This simple three-minute body scan invites you to notice physical sensations and emotions with kindness and curiosity, building awareness that helps you to respond thoughtfully rather than react automatically.

Here are the steps to follow:

1. Sit comfortably with your feet firmly grounded on the floor.

2. Close your eyes or soften your gaze and bring your attention to your natural breath. Notice the rhythm of your inhales and exhales without trying to change them.

3. Slowly guide your focus through your body, starting at the top of your head and moving down toward your toes.
4. As you scan, notice any sensations you feel, such as tightness, fluttering, heaviness, warmth, or numbness.
5. If emotions arise, quietly name them, for example, anxiety, frustration, or tiredness, without judgment or the need to fix anything.
6. Allow all these sensations and emotions to be as they are, offering them acceptance and space.
7. When your mind wanders, gently bring your focus back to your breath or bodily sensations.

Apart from noticing the early signs of stress and emotions, this practice also gives you a moment to pause and choose how to respond, creating emotional self-leadership at its core.

Breath Regulation: Calming the Nervous System

Your breath is a powerful and accessible tool for calming your nervous system and reducing emotional intensity. Because breathing is both automatic and under your control, consciously shifting your breath patterns can quickly signal your brain that it's safe to relax. This helps reduce stress hormones like cortisol, lower heart rate, and even clear mental fog. Below are two effective breathing techniques: diaphragmatic breathing for managing ongoing stress, and box breathing for quick relief during acute anxiety.

Diaphragmatic Breathing for Ongoing Stress:

This technique encourages deep, mindful breaths that fully engage your diaphragm, the muscle below your lungs, helping you move away from shallow chest breathing, which is common during stressful times. Practicing diaphragmatic breathing regularly trains your body to activate your parasympathetic "rest and digest" system, helping you to calm down and focus.

Here's how to do it:

1. Find a comfortable seated or lying position. Place one hand on your chest and the other on your belly to feel the movement.

2. Inhale slowly through your nose for a count of four seconds, focusing on expanding your belly so the hand on your belly rises while the hand on your chest stays relatively still.

3. Exhale gently through your mouth for six seconds, feeling your belly fall as you fully release the air.

4. Repeat this cycle for 6 to 10 breaths, maintaining slow, steady rhythms.

5. Notice any sensations as your body begins to relax and your mind quiets.

6. Use this exercise during moments of sustained stress, such as during a busy afternoon or before falling asleep, to encourage ongoing relaxation.

Box Breathing for Acute Anxiety:

Box breathing is a rhythmic technique that adds breath-holding to both the inhale and exhale phases. This pauses and controls your breath, which can rapidly calm your racing mind or sudden panic by steadying your nervous system and bringing focused attention to the present moment.

These are the easy steps:

1. Sit or stand comfortably with your back straight, shoulders relaxed.

2. Inhale slowly through your nose for a count of four seconds, filling your lungs fully.

3. Hold your breath gently for another four seconds without straining.

4. Exhale slowly through your mouth for four seconds, emptying your lungs completely.

5. Hold your breath again for four seconds before beginning the next inhale.

6. Repeat this cycle at least four times or until you feel calmer.

7. Use box breathing when anxiety spikes suddenly, for example, before a stressful meeting, during moments of panic, or anytime you need a quick reset.

Breath regulation offers an immediate way to calm you emotionally and center your focus. Whether you're managing ongoing stress with diaphragmatic breathing or quieting acute anxiety with box breathing, regular practice builds your capacity to soothe your nervous system naturally.

Cognitive Reframing and Self-Compassion

Perimenopause often brings uninvited shifts in your mood and cognitive function that can result in you being overly critical of yourself. Cognitive reframing is a gentle practice that helps you step back from those negative thought patterns and view your experiences through a more compassionate and realistic lens. When paired with self-compassion, it becomes a powerful tool to reduce your emotional distress and support your mental well-being during this transitional phase.

Steps for reframing and self-compassion include:

- **Notice your automatic negative thoughts:** Become aware of when your mind jumps to extremes or harsh self-judgment. Examples of these can include unrealistic thoughts such as "I'm losing my mind" or "I'll never get this right."

- **Challenge and reframe the thought:** Ask yourself: Is this thought really true? Is there another way to understand the situation that's less extreme and more helpful?

For example, replace "I'm losing my mind" with something like: "Brain fog is common during perimenopause, and I can support myself with tools like reminders and breaks."

- **Add a layer of self-compassion:** Speak to yourself as you would a close friend facing a tough time. Use compassionate statements such as:
    - "This is a moment of difficulty."
    - "Many women experience this during perimenopause."
    - "May I be kind and gentle to myself right now."

Cognitive reframing helps you to develop mental clarity and reduce anxiety, but when paired with self-compassion, you gain even more control over your emotions. Self-compassion helps you understand that your struggles are universal and encourages you to be more patient toward yourself. It helps you tolerate discomfort without shame or frustration, making it easier to care for yourself in challenging moments.

Setting Healthy Boundaries

Setting boundaries is a vital skill for nurturing emotional resilience, especially during the shifts of perimenopause. Boundaries help protect your time, energy, and well-being by creating clear limits around what you want or can handle without guilt or overcommitment. You might feel like you're pushing people away when you set strong boundaries in your life, but they are actually acts of self-respect. Every time you say "no" to something you don't want, you're essentially saying "yes" to something you do want.

When your day is packed, and your emotional energy is running low, it's harder to stay calm and handle stress without snapping or spiraling. Overcommitment can leave you exhausted, irritable, and feeling like even small things hit you harder than they used to. Setting clear boundaries is how you give yourself the space to rest, recharge, and actually respond to life instead of just react. It's the secret to maintaining your resilience.

You don't have to make a big scene or feel awkward about it. Simple, kind, and honest words are all it takes to honor your needs while keeping your relationships intact. Here are a few gentle ways to say what you need without guilt:

- "I appreciate the invite, but I need to rest tonight."
- "I'm grateful you thought of me, but I can't take that on right now."
- "I'm focusing on my health this week, so I'll have to say no."
- "I need to prioritize some downtime, so I won't be available for extra tasks."

Remember, saying "no" to others is saying "yes" to yourself and what's really important for you, which is essential for emotional stability.

Setting healthy boundaries is one of the most empowering things you can do for yourself. It helps you honor your limits, protect your emotional energy, and say "enough" before stress takes over. Boundaries give you the space to show up fully for the things that really matter, instead of running on empty. Think of them as the foundation for building the resilience and balance you need to use perimenopause as a true reset, and to thrive beyond it. In Chapter 11, you'll find practical tips for setting boundaries in all areas of your life, so you can protect your energy without guilt.

Developing Emotional Self-Leadership

Emotional self-leadership is about understanding your own inner experience and learning to guide your emotional responses with awareness and intention. It's about building resilience and creating space for choice through gentle, consistent actions. You develop this leadership through four foundational pillars, each one helping you navigate the emotional waves of perimenopause with more clarity and calm, and giving you the tools to fully reset your life during this time.

Self-Awareness

Self-awareness means tuning in to your own feelings, triggers, and physical signals as they pop up throughout your day. A practical way to do this is by keeping a journal or jotting quick notes whenever you notice these moments.

What to track:

- **Shifts in mood:** When do you feel more irritable, anxious, or joyful?

- **Triggers:** These can be specific situations, people, or thoughts that evoke strong emotions.

- **Energy dips:** Are there specific times when fatigue or tension peaks?

- **Patterns:** These can be related to sleep, stress, and nutrition, which often influence your mood.

Over time, you'll create your own early-warning system, helping you understand when you tend to react with big emotions. This allows you to step in with coping tools before your emotions boil over. The more you practice noticing your emotions and what's happening around you, the more you gain the power to guide your experience instead of being swept along by it.

Consistent Regulation Habits

Awareness is just the first step. To lead your emotions, you need to practice regulation tools regularly. These techniques help quiet your nervous system and strengthen the pathways in your brain that support calmness and mental clarity, so you can respond to challenges with more ease.

Examples can include:

- breathing exercises, such as diaphragmatic or box breathing, that we discussed earlier in this chapter
- grounding techniques, like feeling your feet on the floor or focusing on physical sensations
- gentle mindfulness pauses during the day

Even spending just a minute each day on these practices can strengthen your brain's ability to handle stress. Over time, these habits become automatic, helping you stay balanced even when hormones fluctuate or life feels demanding.

Intentional Emotional Goals

Setting purposeful, value-based emotional goals gives you direction in your daily choices and interactions. These goals don't need to be big or ambitious. Instead, focus on small but meaningful shifts that are in line with what matters most to you.

Sample goals can include:

- "I will pause before responding during conflict."
- "I will bring patience and kindness into my daily conversations."
- "I will create at least one meaningful moment of connection each day."

By anchoring your focus in these intentions, you guide yourself away from reactive patterns and toward conscious, values-driven choices. This helps you to shape your emotional landscape in ways that support your well-being.

Supportive Rituals

Supportive rituals are simple, repeatable practices that help calm your emotions and bring a sense of stability when hormonal shifts make things feel unpredictable.

Examples can include:

- Five minutes of morning mindfulness to set a calm tone for the day.
- A midday breath or grounding check-in to reset nervous system balance.
- Evening journaling to reflect on emotional wins and challenges.
- A weekly Sunday ritual of reviewing your journal and setting new goals.

When you integrate these small rituals into your day, you build a rhythm that supports you through the changing tides, gently reminding you that emotional self-leadership is an ongoing practice rooted in kindness and consistency.

A Daily Emotional Self-Leadership Routine

Building emotional self-leadership into your day doesn't have to take hours or involve complicated practices. Small, consistent moments of awareness and care can add up to real emotional steadiness and resilience. This simple daily routine brings together self-awareness, regulation, reflection, and goal-setting in manageable steps that fit even your busiest days.

Morning: Awareness Check (Two minutes)

Start your day by gently tuning in to your emotional landscape before the outside world pulls you in. This brief check-in sets a mindful tone for the hours ahead:

1. Find a quiet moment with your morning beverage or a comfortable seat.

2. Close your eyes or soften your gaze and ask yourself: "What am I feeling right now?" Name your primary emotion, whether it's calm, anxiety, tiredness, hope, or something else.

3. Choose one intention to guide your day. This might be a value or quality you want to embody, like patience, kindness, courage, or presence.

Starting your day with this conscious check-in anchors your awareness and primes your mind to respond with intention instead of reactivity.

Midday: Regulation Moment (One minute)

Midday moments can be overwhelming. Taking a short pause helps you recalibrate and restore balance:

1. Pause and bring your attention to your body and breath. Notice any tension or tightness.

2. Choose a quick regulation tool, such as a few deep diaphragmatic breaths, a brief mental reframe of a challenging thought, or grounding by feeling your feet firmly on the floor.

3. Use this moment to reset, leaving behind built-up stress and opening space for calm focus.

This midday pause interrupts emotional buildup, refreshing your nervous system so you can carry on with clearer calmness.

Evening: Reflection (Three minutes)

End your day by reflecting on your emotional journey. This closing ritual builds self-awareness and appreciation for your progress:

1. Write down a moment when you felt steady or calm during the day.

2. Note one challenge or difficulty you encountered. Ask yourself something like, "What triggered it or how did it make me feel?"

3. Capture one insight or lesson you learned about your emotions or coping strategies.

Reflecting on your day encourages self-compassion, shows your growing emotional wisdom, and prepares you for tomorrow's intentional practice.

Weekly: Review and Set an Emotional Goal

Once a week, take a slightly longer pause to see patterns and plan ahead:

1. Review your daily notes or journal to identify recurring emotions, triggers, or successes.

2. Identify what emotional needs or challenges stood out.

3. Choose one specific emotional aim or intention to focus on for the coming week, for example, practicing patience, managing anxiety, or creating connection.

Setting weekly goals turns self-leadership into a dynamic process of learning and growth, helping you make meaningful shifts one step at a time.

Knowing When to Seek Professional Support

While emotional self-leadership gives you essential tools to manage your perimenopause symptoms, there will be times when professional support is needed. Knowing when to reach out for extra help is an important act of self-care and wisdom, not a sign of failure or weakness. Professionals can provide guidance, treatment, and resources that complement your personal practices and make a real difference in your well-being.

When to Consider Professional Support

Seek help if you notice any of the following persistent challenges:

- **Sadness or low mood lasting more than two weeks.** Feeling down for an extended period can indicate depression that may warrant professional care.

- **Anxiety that disrupts daily life.** When worry or panic interferes with your work, relationships, or sleep, expert support can offer relief and coping strategies.

- **Memory problems affecting safety or job performance.** If forgetfulness begins to impact your ability to function safely or competently, a professional evaluation might be necessary.

- **Emotional difficulties that don't improve despite your best self-care efforts.** Some struggles require additional intervention to move forward.

Accepting help is a vital part of emotional resilience. It allows you to build a stronger foundation and access resources tailored to your unique needs.

Types of Professional Help Available

Various types of professionals and programs can support you through perimenopause:

- **Psychologists and counselors:** They provide therapy to help people work through emotional challenges and develop coping skills.

- **Psychiatrists:** These doctors offer medical evaluations and, if needed, prescribe medications for mood or anxiety disorders.

- **Support groups:** Joining a support group connects you with others experiencing similar changes, offering community and shared understanding.
- **Menopause specialists:** They focus specifically on hormonal and life-stage changes, integrating medical and lifestyle approaches.
- If cost or access is a concern, consider:
- Online therapy platforms that offer more affordable sessions.
- Community mental health centers with sliding scale fees.
- Employee assistance programs or school-based counseling services.

Professional support comes in many forms, suited to different preferences and budgets. Exploring options makes quality care accessible and manageable.

Partnering With Your Healthcare Provider

Your primary care doctor or gynecologist is an important partner in your holistic care during perimenopause. Be open about your challenges when you see your doctor. Sharing symptoms related to mood, memory, or anxiety helps them to:

- Customize your medical treatment, including hormone management or medications.
- Coordinate referrals to mental health professionals.
- Suggest lifestyle modifications, nutrition plans, and resources to support overall health.

A collaborative, blended approach in combining medical, psychological, and lifestyle support often creates the most effective and comprehensive care for you.

Tracking Regulation With a Daily Log

Recording your mood, focus, and emotional responses in a daily regulation log turns vague feelings into data you can use. This tool helps you spot triggers, highlight opportunities for improvement, and respond with greater insight.

How to Use the Daily Regulation Log

Complete the log at the end of each day, perhaps after dinner or before bed.

For each entry, note:

Mood (for example, content, irritable, anxious, sad, or motivated)

____

____

____

Focus (for example, sharp, distracted, foggy, or steady)

____

____

____

Emotional triggers (describe situations or interactions that affected you)

____

____

____

Coping strategies used (for example, breathing, reframing, or taking a walk)

Overall sense of energy or well-being (for example, high, medium, or low)

Once a week, read through your entries to look for patterns: Do certain events consistently bring anxiety? Does regular mindfulness practice boost morning focus? Use these insights to adjust your habits or reach out for support when symptoms persist.

Reflective Journaling for Emotional Leadership

Writing about your mental and emotional experiences encourages deeper understanding and growth. These journal prompts can help you gain insight and build your confidence as your own emotional leader.

What patterns have I noticed about my mood, energy, and memory over the past week?

Which self-regulation strategies worked well, and where did I struggle?

When did I feel most like myself, and what conditions allowed that feeling?

What would I like to handle differently next time a challenge arises?

What support am I open to asking for, and from whom?

Set aside 10 minutes once or twice a week to write freely in response to these. Reviewing older entries can highlight how far you've come and clarify what works best for you. These practices turn emotional awareness into a steady force for thriving through change.

Final Thoughts

Now that you understand how hormonal shifts impact your mood, memory, and mental clarity during perimenopause, you have the foundation to respond with kindness and confidence rather than frustration or self-doubt. The strategies shared here, from mindful awareness and breath regulation to setting healthy boundaries, offer practical ways to steady your emotions and sharpen your focus amid change. By practicing these skills daily and tuning in to your unique patterns, you can build resilience that supports both your mental health and overall well-being.

This chapter is just the beginning of a reset process designed to help you create lasting balance, so you move through perimenopause with greater ease and preparedness for the next phase of your life.

End of Week 4 Tracker and Journal Prompts

This tracker is designed to help you consolidate the insights and progress you've made over the past two weeks. It combines reflections on your lifestyle pillars, eating, mood, and behavior. Use these journal prompts to deepen your self-awareness, celebrate your progress, and mindfully plan for the weeks ahead.

Six Pillars Reflection and Self-Assessment

In this exercise, you'll explore each of the six pillars more experientially. For each pillar, spend a few moments reflecting on your recent experiences and then brainstorm actionable strategies to better support yourself. This will help you create a personalized plan that respects your unique needs and lifestyle.

Step 1: Reflect on Your Current Experience

For each pillar, briefly describe your recent experience by answering these questions:

Eating: How have my food choices lately affected my energy, mood, or cravings? What foods or patterns have felt nourishing or disruptive?

____

____

____

____

____

____

____

Movement: What types of physical activity or movement have I engaged in? How did they make me feel physically and emotionally?

Stress: How have I noticed stress manifesting in my daily life? What situations or thoughts tend to increase my stress levels?

Sleep: How would I describe the quality of my sleep over the past week? What routines or behaviors have helped or hindered my rest?

____

____

____

____

____

____

____

____

____

Emotions: What emotional patterns or reactions have stood out? Are there particular feelings I notice frequently, or areas where managing emotions feels easier or harder?

____

____

____

____

____

____

____

____

Imbalances: What habits, behaviors, or environmental factors have felt out of sync with my well-being? How do they affect the other pillars?

____

____

____

____

____

____

____

____

Step 2: Brainstorm One Strategy for Each Pillar

For each pillar, write down one small, realistic action you can take to support balance and well-being. Here are some prompts to inspire you:

What small change to my eating might bring steadiness this week?

____

____

____

____

What's one enjoyable or manageable movement I can add or sustain?

____

____

What simple stress-reduction technique could I try when overwhelmed?

What's one adjustment to my bedtime or sleep environment that might improve rest?

What practice or tool could help me better regulate my emotions?

What minor habit or trigger can I gently shift or avoid to reduce imbalance?

____

____

____

____

Step 3: Connect Pillars to Your Life

Briefly describe how these strategies might support the six pillars and create positive effects on the other areas. For example, better sleep can improve emotional resilience and energy for movement. Moving regularly can reduce stress and improve sleep quality.

____

____

____

____

____

____

____

____

____

____

____

Daily Emotional Self-Leadership Practice Tracker

Track your practice of emotional self-leadership habits each day. Mark yes or no and note any reflections. Focus on awareness check-ins, regulation moments, and reflection journaling.

Day	**Morning: awareness check (name your feeling and intention)**	**Midday: regulation practice (breathing, reframing, or grounding)**	**Evening: reflection (steady moment, challenge, or insight)**	**Notes or reflections**
Monday				
Tuesday				
Wednesday				
Thursday				
Friday				
Saturday				
Sunday				

Behavior and Habit Awareness: Identify Your Imbalance Patterns

List two to three habits or routines that pull you off balance, for example, late-night screen use, emotional eating, or skipping meals. For each habit, reflect:

- What usually triggers this habit?

- How does it affect my mood, energy, or other pillars?
- What is one manageable step to interrupt or replace this habit?

1. Habit: ____
    a. Trigger: ____
    b. Impact: ____
    c. Next step: ____
    ____
2. Habit: ____
    a. Trigger: ____
    b. Impact: ____
    c. Next step: ____
    ____
3. Habit: ____
    a. Trigger: ____
    b. Impact: ____
    c. Next step: ____
    ____

Journal Prompts for Deeper Insight

Set aside 10–15 minutes to reflect on any of the following prompts. Write freely and compassionately.

What changes in my mood, energy, or mental clarity have I noticed this past week?

Which self-care habits and tools helped me maintain balance?

What situations or triggers challenged me the most, and how did I respond?

What are 1–2 small changes I want to try next week that feel doable?

How can I cultivate more self-compassion when things feel difficult?

____

____

____

____

____

What progress am I proud of, no matter how small?

____

____

____

____

____

Celebrating Progress

Take a moment to list three wins or positive changes I've experienced this week. These can be anything from small daily habits to shifts in mindset or emotional awareness.

1. ____________________________________

   ____

   ____

2. ____________________________________

   ____

3.

Planning for the Weeks Ahead

What is one emotional or lifestyle intention I want to focus on for the next week?

What support or resources might help me stay on track?

How will I remind myself to practice kindness and patience during this time?

Each mindful choice lays the groundwork for lasting balance, resilience, and ease through perimenopause and beyond. Celebrate your small steps and keep tuning in to what your unique rhythm needs.

Part III:

Deep Dive and Rebuild

(Weeks 5 to 6)

Chapter 7:

Body Systems in Shift—Gut, Bones, Skin, and Libido

Perimenopause affects much more than just your mood, energy, or cognitive function. You may also notice changes in your digestion, bone strength, skin texture, and sexual well-being. These changes can sometimes feel surprising or even unsettling, prompting you to pay closer attention and adjust how you care for yourself.

Think about how you're currently supporting your digestion, bone health, skin, and sexual vitality. Are there areas where you feel confident in your care, and others where you feel more uncertain or challenged?

This chapter invites you to listen deeply to your body's messages and meet these shifts with curiosity and compassion. Understanding how your gut, bones, skin, and libido respond to perimenopause helps you develop a holistic strategy to reset and support your well-being.

Gut Health and the Microbiome

Your gut is one of the most responsive systems during perimenopause. It reacts to hormonal fluctuations, stress, and diet in ways that can feel unpredictable. Many women notice new digestive patterns that feel completely different from what they've experienced previously. A few small changes in how you eat and how you manage stress can bring significant relief.

Hormonal Influence on the Gut Microbiome

Fluctuating levels of estrogen and progesterone during perimenopause have a direct impact on the balance and diversity of your gut bacteria. These hormones help regulate the microbial environment in your gut, but when their levels change, the composition of your gut microbiome may shift as well. Some of the consequences can include (Peters et al., 2022):

- reduced diversity in beneficial bacteria, which can impair digestion and immunity
- increased gut inflammation, contributing to discomfort and digestive symptoms
- altered metabolic health due to the microbiome's role in nutrient absorption and energy regulation

Recognizing that your gut discomfort is linked to hormone shifts helps you approach symptoms with more understanding and motivates gentle adjustments to support your microbiome's balance.

Digestive Changes and Sensitivities

Perimenopause often brings noticeable changes in your digestion and may even make you sensitive to foods you could easily tolerate in the past. You may experience symptoms that seem new or more intense than before, including (Lovink, 2025):

- increased bloating or abdominal discomfort after meals
- fluctuating bowel habits such as constipation or diarrhea

- a general slowing down of digestion, making you feel heavy or sluggish after eating
- emerging or worsening food intolerances, such as sensitivity to lactose, gluten, or certain fibers

These digestive shifts occur because hormonal fluctuations can slow the speed at which food travels through your digestive tract and alter your gut immune responses. This can make your digestive system more reactive, leading to discomfort when consuming foods that previously caused no issues.

Being mindful of your digestion patterns can help you identify which foods or eating habits trigger symptoms. Here are some steps to support your awareness:

- Keep a simple food-and-discomfort diary to track what you eat and how you feel afterward.
- Pay attention to meal timing and portion sizes, as eating too quickly or overeating can worsen symptoms.
- Observe how stress or sleep quality on a given day correlates with digestive comfort.

Understanding these connections guides you toward making mindful dietary choices and lifestyle adjustments that suit your changing needs.

Nutrition to Support Gut Health

Supporting your gut microbiome through mindful nutrition can ease perimenopausal digestive challenges and promote overall well-being. Focus on nourishing the beneficial bacteria in your gut and creating an environment that supports balanced digestion. Here are key dietary strategies to promote gut health:

- **Eat fiber-rich foods:** Vegetables, fruits, legumes, and whole grains are excellent sources of fiber. This fiber feeds the beneficial bacteria in your gut, helping them thrive and maintain balance. Aim to include a variety of colorful vegetables and fruits daily to provide diverse types of fiber and plant compounds.

- **Incorporate prebiotic foods:** Prebiotics are specific types of fiber that act as food for your gut bacteria. Foods rich in prebiotics include onions, garlic, leeks, asparagus, bananas, and chicory root. These can help boost the growth of good bacteria, supporting a diverse microbiome.

- **Include probiotic foods:** Probiotics are live beneficial bacteria that add to the health of your gut microbiome. Fermented foods such as yogurt, kefir, sauerkraut, kimchi, and miso are good sources. Enjoy these regularly to help maintain a healthy bacterial balance.

- **Stay hydrated:** Drinking plenty of water supports digestion by helping fiber move smoothly through your digestive tract and preventing constipation. Aim for at least 8 cups of water daily, adjusting based on activity and climate.

- **Limit processed foods and added sugars:** Foods high in processed ingredients, artificial additives, and added sugars can harm the diversity and function of your gut bacteria. Reducing these foods can help decrease inflammation and support a healthier gut environment.

By consistently including these elements in your diet, you create a nurturing environment for your gut microbiome during the hormonal changes of perimenopause.

Lifestyle Practices for Gut Support

Gut health is influenced by what you eat as well as how you live. The connection between your brain and gut, known as the brain-gut axis, means that your stress levels, physical activity, and daily routines play key roles in your digestive function and microbiome health, especially during perimenopause. Here are a few strategies to consider:

- **Manage stress for a healthier gut:** Chronic stress can upset your digestion, slowing your gut and disrupting healthy bacteria. Using stress-relief techniques can help your gut work better and reduce inflammation. Try these approaches:
  - **Breathwork:** Practice deep diaphragmatic breathing or box breathing for a few minutes daily to calm your nervous system.
  - **Mindfulness and meditation:** Even short meditation sessions can reduce stress hormones and promote relaxation.
  - **Take nature breaks:** Spending time outdoors, especially walking in green spaces, lowers stress and supports gut health.
- **Incorporate gentle movement:** Moving your body helps your digestion by keeping things moving in your gut and boosting blood flow. Simple, regular activities work best, like:
  - **Daily walks:** A 10- to 15-minute walk aids digestion and calms the nervous system.
  - **Gentle yoga or stretching:** Helps relieve tension in the abdomen and encourages regular bowel movements.
  - **Breath-focused movement breaks:** Incorporate breathwork into brief movement pauses throughout your day.
- **Other helpful habits:**
  - Focus on good sleep habits to help your gut heal and communicate better with your brain.
  - Try to avoid eating late at night so your digestive system gets a rest.

- Be careful with antibiotics or other medications because they can upset your gut balance.

Adding these simple habits into your daily life creates a gut-friendly environment, helping reduce digestive discomfort and supporting your overall health during perimenopause.

Bone Strength Through Nutrition and Movement

During perimenopause, bone health becomes especially important. As your estrogen levels decline, your bones can lose density more quickly, raising the risk of fractures. But by understanding these risks and taking proactive steps with nutrition and exercise, you can help keep your bones strong and protect your future health.

Understanding Bone Density Loss Risks

Estrogen is key to keeping your bones strong because it helps balance bone breakdown and formation. When estrogen drops, that balance shifts, and your bones start losing density faster than they can rebuild, making them weaker. Here's what to keep in mind (Cauley, 2015):

- Bone loss usually starts quietly in your 40s but speeds up during and after menopause.
- This makes fractures more likely, especially in your hips, spine, and wrists.
- Being aware of this early gives you the chance to take steps now to protect your bones.

Knowing that perimenopause is a critical time for bone health can motivate you to adopt supportive habits before major bone loss occurs.

Nutrition for Stronger Bones

Keeping your bones strong during perimenopause means focusing on nutrients that help build bone and slow loss. Calcium and vitamin D are the most well-known, but magnesium, vitamin K, and other key micronutrients also support healthy bone metabolism. Here's what to include:

- **Calcium:** Calcium is the major mineral found in bones and is essential for maintaining bone strength. Adults generally need about 1,000 mg to 1,200 mg of calcium daily, depending on age and health status (*Calcium*, 2025). Good sources of calcium include:
    - dairy products such as milk, yogurt, and cheese
    - fortified plant-based milks like almond, soy, or oat milk
    - leafy green vegetables such as kale, collard greens, and bok choy
    - nuts such as almonds and seeds like chia and sesame
- **Vitamin D:** Vitamin D helps your body absorb calcium effectively. It can be obtained through:
    - safe sun exposure, about 10–30 minutes several times per week, depending on skin type and location
    - dietary sources like fatty fish, such as salmon and mackerel, and fortified foods
    - supplements, especially in areas with limited sunlight or for individuals with low vitamin D levels
- **Magnesium:** Magnesium contributes to bone structure. Nuts, seeds, whole grains, and green leafy vegetables are good sources.
- **Vitamin K:** Vitamin K supports bone mineralization. You can find it in leafy greens such as spinach, kale, and broccoli.

Here are a few ways to incorporate these micronutrients into your diet:

1. **Include a source of calcium with every meal.** This might be a serving of yogurt at breakfast, a salad with leafy greens for lunch, or sautéed vegetables with dinner.

2. **Add a portion of fatty fish a couple of times a week** to boost vitamin D naturally.

3. **Snack on nuts and seeds** like almonds or pumpkin seeds to increase intake of both calcium and magnesium.

4. **Use fortified plant milks or cereals** if you reduce dairy, ensuring you still get adequate calcium and vitamin D.

5. **Consider a daily vitamin D supplement** after discussing with your healthcare provider, especially during the winter months or when sun exposure is limited.

By consistently including these nutrients in your diet, you help slow bone loss, maintain strength, and reduce your risk of fractures as you move through perimenopause and beyond.

Load-Bearing and Strength Training Exercises

Physical activity is key to keeping your bones strong during perimenopause. When your muscles and bones work against gravity or resistance, they experience mechanical stress, which stimulates bone growth and slows loss. That's why load-bearing and strength-training exercises are so important. Here's why they matter:

- Bones adapt to the forces placed on them. When you move in ways that challenge your skeleton, bone cells respond by increasing density and strength.

- Declining estrogen during perimenopause slows natural bone remodeling, but exercise helps counteract this.

- Strength training builds and preserves muscle mass. Strong muscles support your bones, improve balance, and lower the risk of falls and fractures.

Effective exercises to include in your routine can be:

- **Weight-bearing aerobic activities:** These include walking, hiking, stair climbing, dancing, or jogging. These activities create impact forces that stimulate bone maintenance.
- **Resistance training:** This involves exercises where muscles work against resistance, such as:
    - free weights (dumbbells or kettlebells)
    - resistance bands
    - bodyweight exercises (squats, push-ups, or lunges)

Here are a few simple steps to follow for building a bone-healthy exercise routine:

1. **Aim for at least two sessions per week** focused on strength training, targeting major muscle groups like legs, back, chest, and core.
2. **Start with simple bodyweight exercises** if new to training, such as:
    - **Bodyweight squats:** Stand with feet shoulder-width apart, lower your hips as if sitting in a chair, then stand back up. Perform 10–12 slow, controlled repetitions.
    - **Wall push-ups:** Stand facing a wall, place your hands on the wall at shoulder height and width, lower your body toward the wall, bending your elbows, and then push back to the starting position. Try 8–10 reps.
3. **Progress to light weights or resistance bands** once you are comfortable. Focus on proper form to avoid injury and maximize benefits.
4. **Incorporate weight-bearing cardio** activities, such as walking briskly or taking the stairs daily. Even 10-15 minutes after meals can support digestion and bone health.

5. **Prioritize recovery:** Allow 48 hours between strength sessions for muscle repair and bone adaptation.

6. **Consider working with a trainer** for guidance on safe progression and tailored exercises if you're new to strength training.

When you make load-bearing and strength training a regular part of your routine, you help your bones stay strong, maintain muscle mass, and boost your overall energy and vitality throughout perimenopause.

Lifestyle Factors Affecting Bone Health

During perimenopause, paying attention to lifestyle factors that affect your bone health is key to preserving bone density and reducing fracture risk. Here's what to watch out for:

- **Smoking:** Smoking reduces blood flow to your bones, slows the activity of bone-building cells, and lowers calcium absorption. It also affects estrogen levels, speeding up bone loss. Quitting smoking is one of the most effective ways to protect your bones.

- **Alcohol consumption:** Drinking too much alcohol can weaken bone structure and disrupt calcium balance, while also increasing the risk of falls and fractures. Keeping alcohol to moderate levels helps protect your bone health.

- **Chronic stress and cortisol:** Prolonged stress raises cortisol levels, which speed up bone breakdown and slow bone formation. Using stress management techniques can help protect your bones.

- **Sedentary lifestyle:** Sitting for long periods without movement reduces the mechanical stimulation that helps keep bones strong, which can lead to faster bone density loss.

- **Excessive caffeine intake:** Too much caffeine can interfere with calcium absorption and increase calcium loss through urine. Limiting caffeine helps maintain the balance your bones need.

By making small, consistent choices around these factors, you can have a big impact on your bone health as your body navigates the hormonal changes of perimenopause.

Gentle Skin Care for Changing Needs

During perimenopause, declining estrogen can change the way your skin feels and works. You might notice it becoming drier, thinner, or more sensitive. Adjusting your skincare routine with gentle, supportive habits can help keep your skin healthy and comfortable during this transition.

Structural and Functional Skin Changes

As estrogen levels drop, your skin produces less collagen, the protein that keeps it firm and elastic. This decrease can lead to:

- thinner skin layers, making skin more fragile and prone to injury
- loss of moisture and natural oils, resulting in dryness and flakiness
- slower wound healing and increased sensitivity to environmental factors

These changes leave your skin more delicate, so it benefits from gentle care that focuses on hydration and strengthening its natural barrier. Noticing these shifts lets you tweak your routine to effectively protect and nourish your skin.

Signs of Increased Sensitivity

During perimenopause, your skin might react differently to products and environmental conditions. Common signs include:

- redness or blotchiness appears more easily
- itchiness or irritation from products you previously tolerated well
- sensitivity to harsh cleansers, exfoliants, or fragranced skincare

Supportive Skincare Routines

Focus on keeping your skin well-hydrated and supporting its natural protective barrier as the base of your daily routine:

- **Gentle cleansing:** Use mild, fragrance-free cleansers that clean without stripping moisture. Wash with lukewarm water instead of hot water.
- **Moisturizing:** Apply creams or lotions rich in ceramides and humectants like hyaluronic acid to lock in hydration and strengthen the skin barrier.
- **Sun protection:** Use a broad-spectrum sunscreen with at least SPF 30 every day, even on cloudy or indoor days, to prevent further collagen breakdown and sun damage.
- **Antioxidants:** Incorporate serums containing antioxidants such as vitamin C to support collagen production and protect against environmental stressors.
- **Avoid over-washing:** Limit cleansing to twice daily to preserve natural oils and avoid dryness.

Mindful Lifestyle and Nutrition to Nourish Skin

Skin health isn't just about what you put on your face. It's also affected by what you put into your body, for example:

- **Hydrate:** Drink enough water throughout the day to support skin moisture. Aim for at least eight cups, adjusting based on activity and climate.

- **Eat omega-3-rich foods:** Include fatty fish like salmon, flaxseeds, walnuts, and chia seeds to help maintain skin elasticity and reduce inflammation.

- **Manage stress:** Practice regular stress reduction techniques, as stress can accelerate skin aging and sensitivity.

- **Get quality sleep:** Sleep encourages skin repair and regeneration, so prioritize consistent, restful sleep each night.

- **Limit sun exposure and avoid smoking:** Protect your skin from ultraviolet rays by wearing protective clothing and avoiding peak sun hours. Smoking damages collagen and accelerates premature aging, so quitting or reducing is beneficial.

Adapting your skincare routine with simplicity, hydration, and protection helps soothe sensitivity, maintain elasticity, and keep your skin feeling healthy and supported through perimenopause and beyond.

Supporting Libido and Sexual Well-Being

Changes in sexual desire and comfort during perimenopause are common, and they're shaped by a mix of biological shifts, emotional factors, and daily stressors. When you understand what's contributing to these changes and begin using supportive, gentle practices, you can maintain a fulfilling sexual life and nurture your overall well-being.

Understanding Libido Changes During Perimenopause

Fluctuating estrogen and testosterone levels can naturally lower your sexual desire during perimenopause. When estrogen drops, you may also experience vaginal dryness or discomfort, which can make intimacy feel physically challenging or even painful at times. On top of the physical changes, emotional shifts like mood swings, higher stress, fatigue, or feeling less connected to your body can all influence how interested you feel in sex.

When you understand that these changes are a normal part of this phase instead of a personal failing, you can treat yourself with more compassion. This awareness also makes it easier to have open, honest conversations with your partner about what you need, what feels comfortable, and how you can stay connected in ways that honor both of you.

Helpful Approaches to Support Sexual Health

Physical comfort during intimacy is essential for maintaining desire, confidence, and connection. During perimenopause, your body may need a little extra support, and that is completely normal. Here are some practical, approachable ways to ease the most common challenges you might experience during this time:

- **Use lubricants and moisturizers:**
    - Choose water-based lubricants to reduce friction and discomfort during sex.
    - Regularly apply vaginal moisturizers to maintain tissue hydration and elasticity.
    - Avoid products with irritants or fragrances that may increase sensitivity.
- **Practice pelvic floor exercises:** Strengthening your pelvic floor muscles can help to improve blood flow, sensation, and muscle tone in your genital area. Here are a few easy steps to do Kegel exercises:
    - Identify your pelvic floor muscles by trying to stop urine flow midstream.

- Tighten these muscles, hold for five seconds, then relax for five seconds.
- Repeat 10–15 times per session, several times a week.

- **Nutritional support:** Zinc and vitamin D contribute to hormone production and sexual function. Include zinc-rich foods such as nuts, seeds, legumes, and seafood, and maintain adequate vitamin D levels through sun exposure or supplementation.

Emotional and Psychological Well-Being

As we've already discussed, perimenopause can have a big impact on your emotional and mental health, which can affect your sexual desire and satisfaction. Support your sexuality by:

- **Practicing open communication:**
  - Share your needs, concerns, and changes with your partner honestly and lovingly.
  - Explore new ways to connect physically and emotionally. This strengthens your relationship and promotes comfort.
- **Using mindfulness and stress management:**
  - Techniques such as focused breathing, meditation, or guided imagery help you stay present and relaxed during intimacy.
  - Reducing anxiety about performance or physical changes can deepen pleasure and connection.
- **Seeking therapy:**
  - If emotional or relationship challenges arise, professional guidance can provide tools and a supportive space to work

through them, enhancing both personal and shared experiences.

Lifestyle Factors That Enhance Sexual Vitality

Physical well-being can also greatly influence your libido and sexual function. Incorporate these habits to support your intimate health:

- **Regular physical activity:** Exercise improves energy, circulation, mood, and body confidence, all of which enhance sexual desire.

- **Prioritize restful sleep:** Quality sleep supports hormone regulation and energy levels, reducing fatigue that can dampen libido.

- **Manage stress:** Implement relaxation techniques and balance work-life demands to reduce chronic stress which can decrease sexual interest.

- **Limit alcohol and avoid smoking:** Excess alcohol can impair sexual response. Smoking restricts blood flow, contributing to reduced sexual function. Cutting back or quitting supports hormonal and vascular health.

By understanding and embracing these holistic strategies, you can boost your sexual health through perimenopause, create a deeper connection with your partner, and find confidence in the bedroom.

Integrating System Health Through the Six Lifestyle Pillars

Your gut, bones, skin, and libido all benefit from the six lifestyle pillars working together. These pillars create a unified approach to self-care during perimenopause:

- **Eating:** Nourishes your gut bacteria, strengthens bones, supports skin health, and balances hormones.

- **Movement:** Stimulates digestion, maintains bone density, boosts circulation for skin, and enhances sexual vitality.

- **Stress management:** Reduces inflammation affecting gut, bones, skin, and libido, while calming the nervous system.

- **Sleep:** Supports tissue repair, hormone balance, mental clarity, and emotional well-being.

- **Emotional regulation:** Builds resilience, reduces cortisol, and promotes healthier physical responses.

- **Addressing imbalances:** Small behavior changes improve all systems by restoring balance and reducing strain.

When these pillars are practiced consistently, they work together to support your body holistically, making care simple, effective, and sustainable.

Reflecting on Your Six Pillars and Body Systems

Use this worksheet to explore how your current habits support your gut, bones, skin, and libido through the six lifestyle pillars.

Eating: What are three ways my current diet supports my gut, bones, skin, or hormonal health?

1. ______________________________

   ____

   ____

2. ______________________________

   ____

   ____

3. ____

____

____

Movement: How does my current physical activity routine benefit multiple body systems? List any exercises or activities I enjoy that support digestion, bone strength, skin circulation, or sexual vitality.

____

____

____

____

____

____

____

Stress management: What stress management techniques do I currently use? How have they helped my physical or emotional well-being during perimenopause?

____

____

____

____

____

____

____

Sleep: How do my sleep habits, and how rest or lack of it, affect my energy, skin health, and emotional regulation?

Emotional regulation: What practices helps me manage my emotions and reduce physical symptoms of stress?

Addressing imbalances: Identify one small behavior that, if changed, could positively impact more than one system, including your gut, bones, skin, or libido.

____

____

____

Setting Integrative Self-Care Goals

Create simple goals that address multiple systems by working through the six pillars.

Choose one small goal related to eating that supports gut, bone, skin, or hormonal health:

____

____

____

____

Choose one small goal related to movement that benefits multiple body systems:

____

____

____

____

____

Pick a stress reduction or emotional regulation practice to add or deepen:

____

____

____

Identify one sleep habit I can improve to promote restoration:

____

____

____

What's one imbalance or behavior I want to gently adjust for overall wellness?

____

____

____

How will I remind myself to practice these goals consistently?

____

____

____

____

Remember, nurturing your gut, bones, skin, and libido is a journey that flows naturally when you incorporate the six lifestyle pillars. Be patient and kind with yourself as you move forward, knowing that every mindful choice contributes to your overall well-being and resilience during perimenopause and beyond.

Final Thoughts

Perimenopause is a time of significant change: physically, emotionally, and hormonally. Understanding how your gut, bones, skin, and libido respond to these shifts empowers you to care for yourself with intention and kindness. By embracing the six lifestyle pillars as your foundation, you create a sustainable and integrative approach that supports your whole body and mind.

Trust in your ability to listen to your body and adapt as you go. Your journey through perimenopause is an opportunity not only to reset but also to thrive in new and meaningful ways.

Chapter 8:

Partnering with Hormones, Medical Options and Building Your Support Team

By now, you've likely gotten used to the subtle changes in your body. Perhaps a sudden heat wave, nights disrupted by sweat, or mood swings don't catch you off guard in the same way they used to. You understand that your body is navigating a new phase, and you want to understand what's happening, what options you have, and how to feel empowered during this transition. You want to know how to make the most of this time so that you can truly reset your lifestyle to thrive in the future.

This might make you wonder about hormone therapy, supplements, who to trust with your care, or even if alternative treatment options would work for you. If these are the things that fill your mind, this chapter is designed for you: to help you make informed choices, build a trusted support team, and partner confidently with your hormones for a healthier, more balanced life.

Navigating perimenopause doesn't have to feel like a solo journey. Here, you'll find clear information about medical and lifestyle options, guidance on choosing professionals attuned to your needs, and tools to advocate for yourself effectively. As you read, reflect on your unique experience and what support feels right for you. With knowledge and collaboration, you can move forward with confidence and grace and truly use this time as a reset for future happiness.

Understanding Hormone Therapy and Supplements

Navigating perimenopause often involves exploring medical options to manage symptoms. Hormone replacement therapy and various supplements can offer relief, but it's important to understand their benefits, risks, and how to approach conversations with your healthcare provider confidently. This knowledge helps you make informed decisions that align with your health goals and personal circumstances.

Overview of Common Hormonal Symptoms and When to Seek Medical Advice

Before we get into different treatment options, let's first focus again on the common symptoms you might experience. Perimenopause can bring a range of symptoms, some mild and manageable, others more severe and needing prompt care. Use this guide to help you identify when you can ride it out and when you should urgently consult your healthcare provider (*Perimenopause*, 2025).

Common symptoms to keep an eye on:

- hot flashes and night sweats
- mood fluctuations such as irritability or mild anxiety
- sleep disturbances like difficulty falling asleep or waking at night
- vaginal dryness or mild discomfort
- changes in libido or sexual response
- mild weight gain or changes in body composition

- mild memory lapses or difficulty concentrating

These symptoms are often part of the natural transition and can usually be managed with lifestyle changes, self-care, and, if needed, medical guidance.

Because some of these symptoms can also be mistaken for stress or other psychological concerns, it's important to seek a qualified healthcare professional who can help with a proper evaluation and differential diagnosis.

Symptoms that require more urgent medical attention might include:

- severe mood changes such as intense depression, suicidal thoughts, or panic attacks

- heavy or irregular vaginal bleeding that is new or significantly different

- sudden, severe headaches or visual changes

- chest pain, shortness of breath, or unexplained swelling (could be signs of cardiovascular issues)

- persistent pelvic pain or unusual vaginal discharge

- significant memory loss or cognitive decline affecting daily functioning

- symptoms causing safety concerns, such as severe dizziness or falls

If you experience any of these symptoms, contact your healthcare provider as soon as possible for an evaluation and possible care.

Hormone Therapy Basics

You've probably heard the words hormone replacement therapy (HRT) many times before, and perhaps had other women tell you their stories of taking the wrong medication, or come across women who deeply regret not using HRT to manage their symptoms. Deciding to use HRT is a deeply personal decision, and one that should be taken under the expert advice from your healthcare professional. If done correctly, it's nothing to fear.

In simple terms, HRT essentially replaces declining estrogen and progesterone levels in your body, and with that, reduces symptoms such as hot flashes, night sweats, mood swings, and vaginal dryness (Harper-Harrison et al., 2024). HRT comes in different formulations, including pills, patches, gels, creams, and vaginal rings, allowing your provider to adapt the treatment to your individual needs and preferences.

Key points to consider about HRT include:

- Timing matters: The sooner you start therapy, the more your body will benefit, and the lower certain risk factors may be.

- Benefits can go beyond symptom relief and extend to supporting bone density and cardiovascular health.

- Risks vary depending on factors such as your age, the type of therapy you choose, your personal health history, and your family history of conditions like breast cancer or blood clots.

Discussing your personal and family medical history with your doctor will help them develop a treatment plan designed specifically for you.

Addressing Myths and Misconceptions About Hormone Therapy

You might hesitate to consider hormone therapy due to the many myths about this treatment that you might have heard. It's important to separate fact from fear by understanding what HRT actually does and doesn't do:

- **Myth:** Hormone therapy causes cancer.

    - **Fact:** Risks vary by individual factors such as therapy type, duration, personal health, and family medical history. For many women, the benefits outweigh the potential risks, especially when the therapy is appropriately managed.

- **Myth:** Hormone therapy should be started only after menopause.
    - **Fact:** Starting therapy closer to the onset of perimenopause often provides better symptom control and reduces some of the potential risks.

- **Myth:** Natural or bioidentical hormones are always safer.
    - **Fact:** "Natural" doesn't guarantee safety or efficacy. All hormone therapies should be prescribed and monitored by healthcare professionals.

Talking openly with your doctor about your concerns can help you make informed, balanced decisions about hormone therapy.

Non-Hormonal Medical Options

For some women, hormone therapy isn't the right fit, whether because of health considerations, personal preference, or simply wanting to explore other options first. If you feel that way, you still have choices. Several non-hormonal medications can help relieve specific perimenopausal symptoms (Migala, 2024):

- **Antidepressants (SSRIs/SNRIs):** These are often prescribed for mood changes and hot flashes.

- **Gabapentin:** Originally developed for seizures, it can reduce hot flashes and improve sleep.

- **Clonidine:** A blood pressure medication that may alleviate hot flashes in some women.

Understanding the possible side effects and what you can realistically expect from treatment helps you choose the option that fits you best. These alternatives give you meaningful ways to manage symptoms without using hormones, but it's still important to talk with your doctor before starting anything new. They can guide you through the risks, benefits, and what makes the most sense for your health.

Dietary Supplements and Botanicals

You may find yourself exploring supplements as a way to support hormonal balance or ease specific symptoms. If you decide to go this route, here are some ingredients you'll see most often (Lubeck, 2025):

- **Vitamin D and magnesium:** These supplements support bone health and nervous system function.

- **Omega-3 fatty acids:** These help reduce inflammation and can even support your mood.

Many healthcare professionals encourage you to not rely solely on supplements. They can be helpful, but they work best when paired with supportive lifestyle habits such as balanced nutrition, regular movement, stress management, and good sleep. When you combine these approaches, you create a stronger, more reliable foundation for managing perimenopause and feeling your best.

Preparing for Provider Conversations

Feeling confident and prepared for medical appointments helps you to advocate for your needs. Consulting with your doctor about your symptoms can be a stressful experience, and you may forget some of the symptoms or even details of your family's medical history. This is why I really encourage you to go into the consultation fully prepared:

- Keep a detailed symptom log noting frequency, intensity, and triggers.

- Create a detailed record of your family's medical history, even things that might not be directly related to your symptoms. It's best to give your healthcare provider too much information than leave out something that might be important for your care.

- Write down questions and treatment goals beforehand to cover during the consultation. Questions you may want to ask your doctor can include:

    - What hormonal changes are likely affecting my symptoms?

    - What treatment options are available for managing my symptoms, including benefits and risks?

    - How do you recommend we monitor my health and adjust treatments if needed?

    - Are there lifestyle changes or therapies that could support my hormone health alongside medical treatments?

    - What side effects should I watch for with any prescribed medications or supplements?

    - How does my medical and family history impact my treatment options and risks?

    - Can you explain how hormone therapy would work and what types are most appropriate for me?

    - What non-hormonal treatments might be effective for my specific symptoms?

    - Are there any support services or specialists you recommend I consult?

- Familiarize yourself with common terms and medical options to reduce anxiety and confusion. Don't hesitate to ask your doctor if they use terms that you don't understand.

- Approach your provider as a partner in care, sharing your preferences and concerns openly.

This collaborative approach will help your healthcare professional create a personalized treatment plan and achieve better health outcomes.

Personalizing Hormone Therapy

Hormone therapy isn't a one-size-fits-all solution. What works for another woman might not be as effective for you. That's why it's best to create a personalized plan based on your needs. Your healthcare provider will consider several factors to personalize your therapy, including your specific symptoms, medical history, lifestyle, and personal preferences.

There are multiple options available, each with different benefits and risks. For example, transdermal patches (through the skin) may reduce certain cardiovascular risks compared to oral hormones, while vaginal applications can target local symptoms like dryness with minimal systemic effects.

Key components of personalization include:

- **Type of hormones used:** Combination of estrogen and progesterone, estrogen alone (for women without a uterus), or bioidentical hormones as prescribed.

- **Dosage adjustments:** Starting with the lowest effective dose and modifying based on symptom relief and side effects.

- **Route of administration:** Choosing between oral, transdermal, or local vaginal delivery according to your health profile and symptom focus.

Regular follow-up appointments are essential to monitor your response to treatment, address side effects, and make necessary adjustments. Open and ongoing communication with your healthcare provider about your symptoms, concerns, and preferences ensures that your therapy remains aligned with your evolving needs.

Remember, your active participation in decision-making creates a personalized, flexible approach that respects your body's unique journey through perimenopause and beyond.

Choosing Clinicians and Forming a Support Team

Navigating perimenopause and midlife health challenges works best when you have a supportive healthcare team and a network of people who understand your unique needs and with whom you feel comfortable. Choosing knowledgeable doctors and building your own support system helps you make confident decisions, stick with lifestyle changes, and truly thrive during this transition.

Identifying Hormone-Savvy Professionals

Finding healthcare providers who really understand perimenopause and women's midlife health can make a big difference for you. Look for doctors with specialized training or experience in this area. Gynecologists, endocrinologists, integrative medicine physicians, or menopause specialists are all great options.

Consider these tips when choosing a provider:

- Check credentials and certifications related to women's health and hormonal care.
- Read patient reviews and seek recommendations from trusted sources or other women in your community.
- Ask potential providers about their experience with perimenopause and hormone therapy.
- Choose someone who listens actively, respects your story, and honors your individual health goals.

Incorporating Behavioral and Nutritional Experts

Medical care works best when paired with support for your lifestyle and emotional health. Working with a psychologist, dietitian, or health coach can help you:

- Develop sustainable habit changes related to nutrition, movement, and stress management.
- Manage emotional challenges and cultivate resilience through regulation strategies.
- Adapt nutrition plans that support hormonal balance and symptom relief.

Keeping open, collaborative communication with your health team helps you get integrated, whole-person care, making your journey through perimenopause smoother and more empowering.

Building a Personal Support Network

Beyond your healthcare team, your well-being also grows when you lean on emotional and social support. Family, friends, and peer groups can offer encouragement, understanding, and accountability, and remind you that you don't have to face this alone. Connecting with other women going through similar transitions lets you share ideas, stories, and practical tips, which can be a huge help during challenging symptoms.

Here are a few tips to strengthen your personal network:

- Share your experiences and needs openly with trusted loved ones.
- Seek out perimenopause or women's midlife support groups, either locally or online.
- Celebrate your progress and discuss your challenges to keep you motivated.

Navigating Healthcare Systems and Resources

Healthcare environments and insurance systems can be complex. Being proactive helps you access care efficiently and reduces stress:

- Learn about your insurance coverage, referral requirements, and appointment processes.
- Follow up consistently and keep thorough notes on treatments and outcomes.
- Explore online educational resources and support groups as valuable supplements to in-person care.

Taking charge of your healthcare journey increases your confidence and helps you advocate effectively for your health.

Importance of Regular Health Screenings

During perimenopause, regular health screenings become particularly important to monitor changes and prevent potential complications. Recommended screenings may include:

- **Bone density tests** to assess the risk of osteoporosis and fracture
- **Cardiovascular assessments**, including blood pressure and cholesterol checks
- **Breast exams and mammograms**, based on your age and family history
- **Pelvic exams and Pap smears** for reproductive health monitoring

Staying up to date with screenings will allow your doctor to catch and treat any issues early.

Empowerment in Decision Making and Advocacy

Making all these choices about your health during perimenopause can feel overwhelming, but developing confidence and self-advocacy skills helps you take charge. When you feel informed and heard, you not only make better health decisions but also gain a stronger sense of control over your journey.

Building Knowledge to Inform Choices

Understanding your body, the available treatment options, and the science behind them can help ease fear and give you confidence in your decisions. You can take charge by:

- Seeking information from reputable sources such as trusted medical organizations, peer-reviewed studies, and expert guidelines.

- Asking providers clear questions about the risks, benefits, and alternatives of suggested treatments.

- Using critical thinking to differentiate between marketing claims and scientific facts, and protecting yourself from misinformation.

Being informed gives you more control, so you can choose the care plan that fits your needs, preferences, and values.

Integrative and Complementary Approaches

You may find that combining complementary therapies with your traditional medical treatments helps you manage perimenopause symptoms more effectively. These integrative approaches support the connection between your body and mind, helping you feel more balanced and resilient during this hormonal transition.

Common complementary therapies can include:

- **Acupuncture:** This ancient practice involves inserting fine needles into specific points on the body to stimulate energy flow and promote healing. Acupuncture has shown promise in reducing hot flashes, improving sleep quality, and alleviating mood disturbances during perimenopause.

- **Mindfulness meditation:** Mindfulness techniques cultivate present-moment awareness and acceptance, reducing stress and emotional reactivity. Regular meditation practice can ease anxiety, enhance mood, and improve sleep patterns, all commonly challenged during perimenopause.

- **Yoga and gentle movement:** Yoga combines physical postures, breath control, and meditation to support flexibility, strength, stress relief, and emotional balance. Gentle forms of yoga, tai chi, and qigong are particularly beneficial for promoting relaxation and mind-body connection.

Not every complementary therapy will be right for you. Some herbs or supplements can interact with medications or may not be safe depending on your health conditions. Always let your medical team know about any complementary treatments you're using. This helps to keep your overall care safe and effective.

Preparing for Your Healthcare Appointment

Use this worksheet to organize your thoughts and goals before meeting with your healthcare provider.

List the most pressing symptoms or health concerns I want to discuss:

____

____

____

____

Write down any questions I want to remember to ask during my appointment:

___

___

___

___

___

What are my health and lifestyle goals related to perimenopause and hormone management?

___

___

___

___

___

Are there treatments or approaches I prefer or want to avoid? What boundaries or concerns do I have?

___

___

___

___

___

Building Your Advocacy Skills

Reflect on how you communicate and advocate for your health needs.

Think about a recent healthcare appointment. How comfortable did I feel expressing my needs and concerns?

____

____

____

____

____

What strategies have helped me communicate clearly with providers? What could I improve?

____

____

____

____

____

____

____

____

____

____

____

Write down three affirmations or reminders that empower me to advocate for myself confidently.

1. ____

____

____

2. ____

____

____

3. ____

____

____

Empowerment and Self-Compassion

Take some quiet time to reflect on these prompts and journal your thoughts if you like.

How does learning about my health and treatment options change my feelings about managing perimenopause?

____

____

____

____

____

____

In what ways can I practice kindness and patience with myself during times of uncertainty or when outcomes are unclear?

How can I balance respect for medical expertise with confidence in my own knowledge and preferences?

What support systems or resources could help me feel more empowered and less alone in my health journey?

____

____

____

____

You build empowerment through knowledge, clear communication, and self-compassion. Approach this process with patience and kindness, and celebrate your progress along the way. Every intentional choice you make supports your well-being and helps you navigate perimenopause with confidence and grace.

Final Thoughts

Navigating perimenopause and the health decisions that come with it can feel challenging, but it's also an opportunity to take charge of your well-being. Empower yourself with knowledge, clear communication, and thoughtful advocacy, turning healthcare from a source of stress into a true partnership that meets your unique needs.

Remember, you are the expert on your own body and experience. By actively participating in your care and practicing self-compassion, you build resilience and create a sense of control amid change.

Chapter 9:

Eating With Intention and Joy—Flexible Meals to Reduce Cravings and Sustain Energy

When you're going through perimenopause, eating isn't just about fueling your body anymore. Many times, the snacks you're craving aren't about hunger but rather about comfort, stress, or habit, as we've explored in Chapter 6. Or perhaps you recall in Chapter 4 learning the basics of nutrition and the vital role of protein, fiber, and healthy fats in supporting your hormones and keeping your energy steady.

Now, imagine sitting down to a meal that feels like a celebration rather than a chore. A meal where you're fully present, savoring every bite, feeling nourished and satisfied without guilt or anxiety. Eating with intention and joy is about reclaiming these moments. It's about shifting from rigid rules or just "what to eat" lists to welcoming flexibility, pleasure, and mindfulness into your everyday eating.

Let's explore strategies to help you fully enjoy food, manage cravings with kindness, and create meals that sustain your energy and honor your body's unique rhythms. Try the different techniques we discussed here to discover what works for you and develop your own eating plan. It's time to bring the joy back to your table and support your well-being through every nourishing bite.

Focus on Mindset and Eating Experience

Eating well during perimenopause is about much more than what's on your plate. It's about how you eat and the relationship you create with food. You may find that the hormonal shifts of this time can stir up old patterns of emotional or habitual eating, making it difficult to trust your hunger cues or to feel satisfied.

Mindful eating is a powerful practice that encourages you to slow down, engage all your senses, and savor each bite fully. It's about being present and tuning into how food tastes, smells, feels, and even sounds as you chew. This connection helps you enjoy your food more and helps you to feel full, reducing overeating and leftover cravings.

Beyond the sensory experience, mindful eating opens space to notice your emotions or thoughts around food without judgment. Maybe you recognize a tension melting away with each bite or a quiet urge to eat when stressed or bored. Meeting these feelings with curiosity rather than criticism allows you to gently shift your relationship with food from one of conflict to compassion.

Strategies for Social and Real-Life Eating Challenges

Eating doesn't happen in a vacuum. It's woven into your social life, celebrations, workdays, and travel. During perimenopause, when your body and hunger cues might feel less predictable, navigating these real-world eating situations can sometimes be daunting.

Social gatherings, holidays, and dining out often come with tempting but unfamiliar foods, bigger portions, and distractions that can make mindful eating tough. Instead of striving for perfection, which can fuel anxiety and feelings of failure, embrace flexibility and presence. Allow yourself to enjoy the flavors, aromas, and company with curiosity rather than judgment.

Honoring your hunger and fullness signals in unpredictable environments is a powerful act of self-trust. You might find that eating a smaller portion, savoring one favorite dish, or pausing between bites to assess fullness helps you maintain balance. Remember, it's okay to say "no, thank you" to additional servings or foods that don't feel right in the moment. Setting gentle boundaries is part of honoring your body's needs.

Travel and busy schedules can also disrupt your usual meal patterns, but planning with adaptable snacks and openness to new foods can reduce stress. Use travel or event days as opportunities to experiment with flexibility. Perhaps you can try a small portion of something new or blend a trusted snack with local flavors.

Ultimately, the ability to adapt during social and real-life eating situations with kindness and adaptability creates a joyful, sustainable way of nourishing your body despite life's unpredictability.

Energy Management Through Timing and Intuition

Perimenopause often brings shifts in energy levels throughout the day and month. You might notice familiar patterns like a mid-morning dip in focus, a pronounced 3 p.m. slump, or evenings when cravings intensify. Understanding and working with these bodily rhythms offers a way to manage energy sustainably without rigid meal schedules or restrictive eating.

Tuning into your body's signals and hormonal fluctuations allows you to eat responsively, using food as a tool to smooth out energy highs and lows. This intuitive approach embraces flexibility rather than strict timing, empowering you to honor your unique rhythm daily.

Common energy rhythm patterns during perimenopause include:

- **Mid-morning dip:** Your blood sugar and alertness may decline a few hours after breakfast. A small, protein-rich snack or a hydrating beverage might help you stay focused and steady.

- **Three p.m. crash:** Energy often drops mid-afternoon, triggering cravings for sweets or caffeine. Balancing protein, fiber, and healthy fats in your lunch can help prevent this dip. If it still hits, a mindful, nutritious snack can restore balance.

- **Evening appetite changes:** Some women find their appetite increases or becomes less predictable in the evening. This may reflect hormonal or stress-related shifts. Choose satisfying, nutrient-dense foods that feel comforting but support restful sleep.

Here are a few practical strategies for aligning eating with your energy and intuition:

- **Listen before you eat:** Pause and check in with your hunger and fullness signals. Ask yourself, "Am I truly hungry or looking to manage an energy slump or emotion?"

- **Flexible meal timing:** Rather than strict clock-based meals, eat when your body genuinely signals need, adapting portion sizes or food types accordingly.

- **Emphasize balanced nutrient combinations:** Ensure protein, fiber, healthy carbs and fats are present, especially at meals preceding known energy dips.

- **Hydrate regularly:** Sometimes fatigue or hunger signals can mask mild dehydration. Having a glass of water supports your metabolism and energy.

- **Adjust for hormonal cycles:** Some days or weeks may require more frequent snacks, lighter meals, or increased comfort foods. Honor these phases without judgment.

Consider keeping a simple energy and eating journal for a week. Jot down times when your energy dips or cravings arise and note what you ate around those moments. Over time, you'll identify patterns unique to your body's rhythms, empowering you to make intentional, supportive choices.

Craving Science 2.0: Decoding What Your Body Is Asking For

Cravings can feel like mysterious urges that derail your best intentions, but decoding the physiology behind them offers clues to what your body truly needs. Moving beyond emotional eating (explored in Chapter 6), it helps to understand how cravings often relate to specific nutritional or sensory needs, hormonal shifts, and even stress responses during perimenopause.

Recognizing what different cravings tell you will help you to respond nutritively rather than reactively, building a gentler, more effective approach to eating and satisfaction, for example:

- **Salt cravings:**
  - might indicate adrenal fatigue or low sodium due to sweating or stress
  - could reflect the body's need for electrolyte balance, especially if you're active or dehydrated
- **Sugar cravings:**
  - often linked to blood sugar dips or energy slumps (like the 3 p.m. crash)
  - may signal a need for quick energy, but refined sugars can worsen the cycle
  - can also stem from brain chemistry changes involving serotonin and dopamine regulation during hormonal shifts
- **Crunchy cravings:**
  - might suggest a desire for sensory stimulation or oral satisfaction

    - could also reflect tension or the need for distraction or mindfulness

- **Fat cravings:**
    - often relate to the body's need for essential fatty acids that support hormone production, brain health, and mood
    - healthy fats provide lasting satiety and help stabilize blood sugar

- **Caffeine cravings:**
    - may reflect fatigue or adrenal stress, but can contribute to anxiety or disrupt sleep if overused

Next, let's look at ways to interpret your cravings thoughtfully:

- When a craving hits, pause to ask yourself:
    - Am I physically hungry, or is this craving tied to emotion or habit?
    - What specific sensation or feeling is underlying this urge?
    - Can I nourish this need with a balanced option or mindful alternative?

- Experiment with different responses:
    - For a salt craving, try adding olives, pickles, or a small broth-based soup.
    - When sugar beckons, choose naturally sweet options like fresh fruit combined with nuts or yogurt.
    - If crunch is desired, try raw vegetables, roasted chickpeas, or air-popped popcorn.

- Notice how your body and mind respond. Over time, this curious attention can reduce the intensity and frequency of unhelpful cravings.

Understanding the layers beneath cravings, such as nutritional, emotional, sensory, and hormonal, helps you move from impulse to insight. You shift from being pulled by cravings to responding with kindness and knowledge, turning eating into an act of nourishment and wholeness.

Gentle Nutrition: The 20% That Makes 80% Difference

During perimenopause, overhauling your entire diet can feel overwhelming and hard to stick with. Instead, focus on small, key nutritional habits that give you the biggest benefits. The 80-20 rule is a simple way to make lasting change without adding pressure or taking the joy out of eating.

Here's how it works: aim to nourish your body with hormone-supporting, healthful foods most of the time (about 80%) and give yourself flexibility and enjoyment for the remaining 20%.

This approach is all about balance. It helps you make mostly mindful, nourishing choices while still honoring cravings, social events, and the simple pleasure of food without guilt.

Key benefits of the 80-20 mindset include:

- **Sustainability:** It's easier to maintain long-term without feeling deprived.
- **Flexibility:** It adapts to social life, mood, and changing needs.
- **A positive relationship with food:** It reduces guilt and obsessive thinking about eating.
- **Encourages mindful choices:** It supports awareness and intentionality rather than restriction.

By embracing the 80-20 rule, you create space for joyful, nourishing eating that fits your life and supports your hormonal balance naturally.

Eating for Energy: Your Personal Fuel Formula

Everyone's energy needs and eating preferences differ, especially during perimenopause, when hormonal changes can affect your appetite, digestion, and metabolism in unique ways. Instead of chasing a one-size-fits-all plan or aiming for perfection, tuning into your personal fuel formula lets you honor your body's natural rhythms and build sustainable eating habits that support your energy and well-being.

This approach encourages you to notice when and how you feel most fueled throughout the day. Understanding your own patterns helps you adapt meals and snacks to fit your lifestyle and energy flow, making eating feel easier, more satisfying, and less frustrating.

Three of the most common energy profiles are:

- **Protein-first morning person:**
  - You feel best starting the day with a hearty, protein-rich breakfast like eggs or Greek yogurt.
  - Skipping or delaying breakfast often leads to energy dips or overwhelming hunger later.
  - Your meals throughout the day benefit from steady protein to maintain focus and stamina.
- **Small, frequent meal person:**
  - You prefer eating smaller portions more often to avoid energy crashes or digestive discomfort.
  - Frequent snacks balanced with protein, fiber, and healthy fats keep your mood and blood sugar steady.
  - Light meals support your digestion and provide consistent nourishment.

- **Hybrid eater:**
    - You adapt between larger meals and smaller snacks depending on the day's activity, mood, or hormonal flux.
    - You benefit from listening closely to hunger cues and easing up or eating more based on your body's signals.

Flexibility and variety are key in your approach.

To help you identify your own energy profile, ask yourself questions like:

- When do I feel hungriest or most energetic during the day?
- How does skipping or delaying meals affect my mood and focus?
- Do I prefer more structure or flexibility in my eating routine?
- How do different foods and portion sizes make me feel physically and emotionally?

Once you understand your energy profile, you can adjust your meals accordingly, for example:

- **Protein-first morning person:** Start with eggs and veggies, add nuts or cheese for snacks, and balance lunch and dinner with lean proteins and colorful plants.
- **Small, frequent meal person:** Keep protein-rich snacks (like hummus with veggies or nut butter with fruit) handy and opt for balanced mini-meals throughout the day.
- **Hybrid eater:** Practice mindful checking in on hunger, embracing flexibility, and preparing easy, quick options to sustain energy as needs fluctuate.

This personalized approach honors your body's wisdom, supports steady energy, and reduces pressure to "get it right." Eating for energy creates kindness toward yourself and sustainable eating habits during perimenopause.

The Calm Kitchen: Environment's Role in Appetite and Eating Quality

The environment where you eat plays a surprisingly powerful role in how and what you eat. Lighting, noise, clutter, and even your mindset before a meal can influence hunger signals, digestion, cravings, and satisfaction. During perimenopause, when your body may already feel more sensitive or unsettled, creating a calm eating environment can help you reconnect with your natural appetite rhythms and enjoy food more fully.

Let's look at a few ways your eating environment affects appetite and digestion:

- **Lighting:** Soft, natural light encourages relaxation and mindfulness, while harsh or flickering lights can raise stress and disrupt focus on eating.

- **Noise:** Loud or distracting sounds may encourage hurried or mindless eating, while quiet or soothing sounds promote slower, more attentive meals.

- **Clutter:** A tidy, inviting eating space reduces mental clutter and distractions, supporting calm, focused eating.

- **Pace:** Rushing meals often leads to overeating as your brain doesn't register fullness in time; slowing your pace allows better digestion and satisfaction.

Simple micro-habits to create a calm kitchen and mindful eating experience include:

- **Take three calm, deep breaths before sitting down:** This helps transition yourself from busy thoughts to food awareness.

- **Unplug from screens and phones:** Removing distractions helps you tune into hunger and fullness cues.

- **Engage your senses intentionally:** Notice your food's colors, texture, smells, and flavors.

- **Create pleasant rituals:** Lighting a candle, playing soft music, or setting the table nicely can turn meals into nurturing moments.

By crafting a calm, inviting eating space, and slowing down your pace, you create a supportive environment to strengthen your mindful eating practices. This mindful atmosphere helps balance your appetite, reduce impulsive cravings, and deepen the joy and satisfaction found in each meal.

Flexible Hormone-Balance Meal Templates

Eating with intention during perimenopause means combining nourishing foods in ways that balance hormones, reduce inflammation, and support your emotional well-being. Flexible meal templates make meal planning easy and fun, letting you mix and match ingredients to suit your taste, cravings, and lifestyle. These templates focus on simple, satisfying combinations designed to address your changing needs.

The Hormone-Balancing Plate

This classic meal structure centers on steady protein, fiber-rich vegetables, and healthy fats to stabilize your blood sugar, support your hormone production, and keep you satisfied.

- **Protein:** lean meats, fatty fish, legumes, eggs, or tofu

- **Vegetables:** a variety of colorful, fiber-rich veggies like leafy greens, cruciferous vegetables, and bell peppers

- **Healthy fats:** olive oil, avocado, nuts, or seeds

- **Optional carb:** serving of whole grains or starchy vegetables for sustained energy

Eating With Joy: Rediscovering Pleasure, Comfort, and Connection

Food should be a source of pleasure, comfort, connection, and tradition. During perimenopause, when your body and emotions are shifting, rediscovering joy in eating can nourish your body and your spirit.

It's important to enjoy what you eat to have a healthy relationship with food. When you engage your senses and savor flavors, textures, and aromas, you invite relaxation and satisfaction. This mindful enjoyment helps you to regulate your appetite, reduce your cravings, and lower your stress hormones like cortisol, which can otherwise disrupt your metabolism and mood.

Ways to bring joy back to your eating experience can include:

- **Engage your senses fully:** Notice the vibrant colors on your plate, the aroma of spices, the crunch or creaminess in each bite.

- **Eat without distractions:** Turn off screens or put away devices to truly focus on your meal.

- **Savor slowly:** Take smaller bites, chew thoroughly, and pause between bites to notice fullness and flavor.

- **Celebrate food traditions:** Prepare family recipes or seasonal dishes that connect you to your heritage and bring comfort.

- **Cook with intention:** View meal preparation as caring for yourself, experimenting with ingredients and recipes that excite you.

- **Share meals:** Eating with friends or family fosters connection and joy beyond the food itself.

Finding pleasure, comfort, and connection in what you eat supports your body and your emotional resilience during perimenopause. These positive eating rhythms help you feel grounded, nourished, and balanced, day by day.

Mini Habit Builder and Reflection

As you explore flexible eating through this chapter, take a moment to reflect on how your body wants to be fed right now.

What new awareness have I gained about my energy rhythms, cravings, or food enjoyment?

____

____

____

____

____

What small changes can I make this week to eat more mindfully or joyfully?

____

____

____

____

____

How can I show myself kindness if things don't go perfectly?

____

____

____

____

____

____

Remember, gentle observation and small, consistent upgrades build lasting habits rooted in self-trust and pleasure, not pressure.

Sensory Exploration Meal

Choose one meal or snack this week to eat as a sensory exploration experience. The goal is to slow down and engage fully with your food's qualities to enhance satisfaction and awareness:

- Find a quiet, comfortable space without distractions.
- Before you begin, take a few deep breaths to center yourself.
- As you eat, focus on each sense:
  - **Sight:** notice colors, shapes, and presentation
  - **Smell:** inhale the aromas deeply
  - **Touch:** feel the textures between your fingers or on your tongue
  - **Taste:** take small bites, savor all flavor nuances
  - **Sound:** notice any crunch or subtle noises as you chew

When you're done, reflect on your experience:

Which sense did I connect with most fully?

____

____

How did slowing down affect my hunger or fullness cues?

____

____

____

____

Did I notice flavors I usually miss when eating quickly?

____

____

____

Craving Check-In and Response Plan

Use this exercise to bring curiosity and kindness to your next craving, rather than reacting automatically. When a craving arises, pause and ask:

What am I feeling right now emotionally and physically?

____

____

____

Is this craving for a specific taste, texture, or comfort?

Rate my hunger on a scale of 1 (not hungry) to 10 (very hungry).

Identify one nourishing option or comforting non-food activity that could meet the craving or underlying need. Examples can include herbal tea, a brisk walk, a few nuts, or deep breathing.

Choose to act on the option and reflect on how my body and mind feel afterward.

Once you're done, reflect on what you discovered about yourself and your craving:

What was easier or harder about responding intentionally?

How did this practice affect my cravings or mood?

What new strategies or comforts might I add to my toolkit?

Final Thoughts

Perimenopause is a unique journey that invites you to listen more deeply to your body, adapt with compassion, and reclaim joy in the everyday act of eating. This chapter has guided you beyond the what of nutrition into the heart of how to nourish yourself with intention, flexibility, and pleasure.

Remember, there is no perfect meal plan that fits every day or every body. Your evolving needs and rhythms deserve kindness and responsiveness, not judgment or guilt. By tuning into your energy, decoding cravings, creating peaceful environments, and embracing pleasure and connection with food, you build a resilient and joyful relationship with nourishment.

End of Week 6 Progress Map and Lifestyle Check In

This workbook is designed to help you reflect deeply on your journey through perimenopause, track your progress, and create personalized steps forward as you rebuild your health and joy. Use these exercises to integrate insights from recent weeks, celebrate your wins, recognize challenges, and fine-tune your habits to support your body's unique needs.

Body Check-In: Reflection and Priority Setting

Take a moment to reflect on your current sense of health and balance in these key areas:

Digestive health and gut microbiome: How do I feel about my digestion and gut well-being right now?

____

____

____

____

Bone strength and joint health: How strong and resilient do my bones and joints feel?

____

____

____

____

Skin vitality and hydration: What is my skin telling me about hydration and vitality?

____

____

____

____

Libido and sexual well-being: How connected do I feel to my sexual health and pleasure currently?

____

____

____

____

For each area, write a number from 1 (needs attention) to 10 (strong and balanced). Then answer:

Which one or two areas do I feel ready to prioritize in the coming weeks?

____

____

Why do these areas feel important to focus on now?

____

____

____

____

What small, manageable steps could I take to support these priorities?

Medical Empowerment and Support Action Plan

Reflect on your current healthcare and support network:

Who are my healthcare providers and supportive people? This can include doctors, specialists, friends, or coaches.

How well do these people listen, respect my goals, and support my health journey?

Are there any gaps or new resources I would like to explore or add?

Next, set your intentions:

What is one concrete action I will take to enhance or expand my support team?

____

____

____

____

What important question or topic will I bring up at my next healthcare appointment?

____

____

____

____

____

Personalized Nutrition and Energy Blueprint

Choose two or three meal strategies or templates from your recent learning to focus on this week.

Each day this week, jot down:

What did I eat?

____

____

____

How did I feel physically and emotionally before eating?

How satisfied and energized did I feel after the meal?

Did I experience any cravings or energy shifts afterward?

At week's end, reflect on:

Which strategies felt supportive or nourishing?

Did I notice any changes in mood, cravings, or energy?

___

___

___

___

What adjustments might help me next week?

___

___

___

___

___

___

___

Craving and Mood Mapping: Decoding Your Body's Messages

For three to five days, notice your cravings mindfully and journal:

When did the craving occur? Add the time, place, and situation.

___

___

___

___

What type of craving was it? This can include salty, sweet, and crunchy.

How intense was it on a scale of 1 to 10?

What emotion or mood did I experience?

What do I think my body was asking for?

How did I respond to the craving?

What was the outcome? How did I feel afterward?

Afterward, consider:

What patterns or insights emerged about my cravings?

Which responses helped satisfy or reduce cravings effectively?

What new ideas or practices would I like to try?

____

____

____

____

____

____

____

Joyful Eating and Mindful Moments: Creating Personal Rituals

Brainstorm three rituals or mindful habits to enhance pleasure and presence during meals. These can be simple and personalized, for example, lighting a candle, taking mindful breaths before eating, or enjoying meals outdoors.

For each ritual, write:

What is the ritual?

____

____

____

____

____

____

When and how will I practice it?

Try incorporating at least one ritual daily for a week. After that, reflect:

How did this change my experience of eating?

What differences did I notice in my mood, satisfaction, or cravings?

Which ritual felt most nourishing to my body and mind?

Reflect on Your Journey

Take a moment to summarize your journey so far:

What are the most important insights I have gained?

___

___

___

What intentions or commitments will guide my next steps?

___

___

___

___

___

Write a positive affirmation or encouragement to support my ongoing wellness journey.

___

___

___

This workbook marks a meaningful step in your journey to rebuild health with intention and compassion. Remember, progress is a series of small, mindful actions rather than perfection. Use your insights and goals here as a flexible foundation to support your evolving needs through perimenopause and beyond. When challenges come, return to self-compassion and curiosity. Keep listening to your body and adjusting with kindness as you move forward.

Part IV:

Rise and Thrive

(Weeks 7 to 8)

Chapter 10:

Movement That Respects Your Body—Strength, Vitality, and Recovery for Lasting Habits

Movement during perimenopause is less about striving for intense workouts and more about tuning into your body's evolving needs. It's a chance to discover movements that bring you comfort, build resilience, and boost your vitality over time. Earlier chapters laid the groundwork with essential practices like strength training, walking, and gentle mobility. In this chapter, we'll explore how to listen to your body's signals, optimize recovery, and create a joyful, sustainable movement routine that supports you through this transformative phase.

Some days you wake up feeling energized and ready to tackle a brisk walk or a strength session. Other days, your body might feel sluggish, or your joints a little achy, and just the idea of exercise could feel exhausting or even stressful. Maybe you notice that on days when your mood dips or your sleep is off, your motivation to move also drops. These ups and downs are normal during perimenopause. The key is learning how to listen to these signals and adjust your movement, so it supports your well-being rather than adding stress.

Movement shouldn't be seen as a race or a competition, but rather a way to nurture yourself, honor your body, and build lasting energy and resilience. You don't have to do hours in the gym or push through pain to get benefits. Sometimes, the best movement is the one that feels gentle, playful, or calming. Let's explore how you can move through this phase of life with kindness and strength. Try the different techniques we discussed here to discover what works for you and develop your own workout plan.

Training With Your Hormonal Reality: Adaptive Movement for Fluctuating Energy

During perimenopause, shifting hormones can influence your energy, mood, and how your body feels each day. That means your movement needs will change, too. Here's how you can adapt your workouts so you stay consistent, avoid overwhelm, and reduce the risk of injury.

How Hormones Affect Your Movement

Hormonal changes during perimenopause can significantly affect how your body moves and feels. Being aware of these shifts helps you make smarter choices about your workouts:

- **Muscle strength and coordination:** Estrogen supports muscle strength and neuromuscular control. When your levels drop or fluctuate, movements may feel less smooth, and your risk of strains or injuries can increase. Focus on proper form, gradual progression, and mindful movement.

- **Joint health and flexibility:** Estrogen also influences joint lubrication and your connective tissue. You may notice stiffness that limits your range of motion, or periods when joints feel loose or unstable, which can increase injury risk. Pay attention to how your joints feel and modify workouts accordingly. Do gentle mobility exercises when you feel stiff, and stability work when your joints feel loose.

- **Mood, motivation, and focus:** Hormonal shifts affect your neurotransmitters like serotonin and dopamine, which regulate mood and mental clarity. You may feel fatigue, irritability, or brain fog, which can make it harder to stay motivated or concentrate during exercise. Practice self-compassion and adjust your workout plans to support your energy rather than push through frustration.

By understanding how hormones affect both your body and mind, you can move more wisely by nurturing strength, reducing injury risk, and making exercise an enjoyable, supportive part of your perimenopause journey.

Using the Three-Lights System

To decide what kind of movement feels right each day, try this simple three-light system based on how your body and mind feel:

- **Green light days:** You feel energized and ready. Choose strength training, moderate or higher-intensity exercise, or longer walks.

- **Yellow light days:** Your energy is moderate, and your symptoms are mild. Opt for gentle movement, such as mobility work, light strength, slow walks, or restorative yoga.

- **Red light days:** Your energy is low, your symptoms are strong, and you experience aches. Focus on rest or very gentle movements such as deep stretching or breathwork.

This system helps you honor your changing needs and avoid pushing too hard when your body is signaling to slow down. Before exercising, check in with yourself and ask questions like:

- How is my energy right now?

- How do my joints and muscles feel?

- What is my current mood like?

Based on your answers:

1. Use the red, yellow, and green light system to guide your movement intensity.

2. Modify your workout: full effort on green days, reduced effort or gentler activities on yellow days, and rest or very light movement on red days.

3. Pay attention to your movements for signs to pause or adjust, like joint pain or dizziness.

4. Keep weekly plans flexible to accommodate varying energy and recovery needs.

This approach helps you stay active without causing burnout or injury.

Movement Scripts for Specific Symptoms

Some symptoms call for targeted types of movement. Here are suggested approaches you can try when certain symptoms are strong:

- **Anxiety spikes:** Use grounding, slow-strength movements, or calming yoga combined with deep breathing.

- **Rage or irritability:** Try expressive, free movements like dancing or shaking to safely release tension.

- **Brain fog:** Engage in repetitive, focused movements such as walking or light strength exercises.

- **Low mood:** Move outdoors with activities like walking in nature paired with breathwork.

- **Headaches:** Opt for gentle neck and shoulder stretches with breath focus. Avoid strenuous workouts.

- **Hot flashes:** Choose slow, cooling movements, such as restorative yoga and gentle stretching in a cool environment.

Adjusting your movement with your hormones and symptoms in mind doesn't have to be complicated. Listening and responding with flexibility, you build a routine that supports your health, respects your body, and keeps you moving in a way that feels good.

Building Resilience Through Rest Cycles

Recovery is more than just taking a day off or getting good sleep. During perimenopause, your body's needs for rest and repair change, and understanding these deeper recovery principles can make a big difference in how your body responds to movement and stress.

Why Recovery Matters More Now

As your hormones fluctuate, your muscles, joints, and nervous system may take longer to bounce back after exercise or stress. Recognizing this helps you avoid overtraining and burnout, which can set back your progress and affect your well-being. Here are a few factors to consider:

- Perimenopausal bodies often require longer recovery windows than before.
- Cortisol, the stress hormone, can interfere with muscle repair and performance if elevated.
- Learning to distinguish productive fatigue (the kind that signals growth) from stress fatigue (which harms progress) is key.

Understanding these factors empowers you to prioritize recovery wisely.

Active Recovery and Micro-Circulation Boosters

Rest doesn't always mean complete stillness. Active recovery can involve gentle movement that encourages blood flow and supports your body's healing. Here are a few examples:

- Use contrast showers by alternating warm and cool water to stimulate circulation.

- Try gentle release techniques such as foam rolling to reduce muscle tightness.

- Incorporate slow, flowing mobility exercises that feel soothing and decrease stiffness.

These practices support better circulation and quicker recovery.

The 48-Hour vs. 72-Hour Rule

Not all recovery days are created equal. Depending on your hormonal state and how you feel, you may need to adjust how much rest you take between workouts:

- On most days, a 48-hour recovery between strength sessions may be sufficient.

- During hormonal lows or higher stress periods, extending recovery to 72 hours can be more beneficial.

Listening to your body and adjusting your rest periods helps you maintain progress without risking injury or exhaustion.

Recovery is Essential for Strength Gains

Recovery should be viewed as a vital part of your training routine, not optional downtime. Without adequate rest, your muscles can't rebuild strongly, and your nervous system can't reset fully.

Prioritize sleep, nutrition, hydration, and effective recovery strategies as foundational to building strength, vitality, and resilience during perimenopause. Learning to recover well ensures that your movement supports your long-term health.

Joint-Friendly Movement for Hormone-Sensitive Bodies

Joint and connective tissue health becomes increasingly important during perimenopause. As your estrogen levels decline, your joints and tendons may feel less stable or more prone to discomfort. Let's look at how you can protect and strengthen these areas through targeted movement.

Why Joint Health Changes During Perimenopause

Estrogen helps keep your joints, tendons, and fascia flexible and resilient. When levels drop, you might notice:

- increased joint laxity or looseness, which can raise injury risk
- stiffness or discomfort in common areas like knees, hips, shoulders, or the lower back
- slower recovery from movement due to connective tissue changes

Being aware of these changes helps you adjust your warm-up and strengthening routines to support joint health.

Warm-Ups Tailored to Hormonal Changes

A thoughtful warm-up is essential to prepare your joints and muscles for any sort of exercise. Focus on gentle, joint-friendly movements that increase blood flow and mobility without strain, such as:

- Perform slow, controlled movements targeting hips, shoulders, spine, and knees.
- Include dynamic stretches such as leg swings, arm circles, and spinal twists.
- Keep the warm-up short and consistent. About three minutes is enough to prime your body.

Prioritizing this warm-up reduces injury risk and promotes smoother movement.

Gentle Prehab: Strengthening Key Areas

Building strength around your vulnerable joints will help to protect them from injury and support your overall daily function. Focus on exercises that target:

- **Knees:** chair sits, wall sits, and mini squats to strengthen the quadriceps and support the joint

- **Hips:** glute bridges, side-lying leg lifts, and hip marches to stabilize the pelvis

- **Shoulders:** wall push-ups, scapular squeezes, and resistance band rows to improve shoulder stability

- **Back:** bird-dogs, plank holds, and dead bugs to enhance core and spinal support

These movements should be done with controlled form, low weight or resistance, and can be incorporated into your routine two to three times per week.

For best results and to ensure these exercises are performed safely and effectively for your individual needs, consider working with a certified personal trainer who can guide and personalize your program.

Fascia-Liberating Movement

Your fascia, the connective tissue surrounding muscles and organs, can become tight or restricted with hormonal shifts. Gentle fascia-liberating techniques help restore your mobility and reduce any tension you may experience, for example:

- Slow, dynamic stretches combined with deep breathing promote fascial flexibility.

- Bouncing or gentle rhythmic movement targets fascia lengthening without strain.

- Gently applying basic foam rolling on major muscle groups aids circulation and fascia health.

Taking care of your joints with hormone-sensitive movement prepares your body for both exercise and everyday activities. These strategies can help you stay active for longer and feel more comfortable in your body.

Building a Nervous-System-Smart Movement Routine

Movement is about more than just your muscles and joints. It also deeply affects your nervous system. Understanding how your body reacts emotionally and physically to movement can help you create routines that calm, energize, or balance your system.

Discovering Your Movement Nervous System Type

Everyone's nervous system responds differently to movement stress. Identifying your nervous system type can guide you to the movements that best support your emotional and physical well-being. Here are three common types:

- The **Burner** tends to have high anxiety and benefits most from grounding, calming movements.

- The **Fader** often experiences low energy and improves with stimulating, rhythmic movement.

- The **Drifter** has inconsistent energy and thrives with a balance of structure and flexibility in movement habits.

Recognizing your type helps you select movement that meets your nervous system's needs.

Using Movement to Regulate Emotions

Movement is a powerful tool for self-regulation. You can harness different kinds of movement for specific emotional needs:

- **Grounding movements:** Heavy lifts, slow and weighted exercises, and steady postures help settle anxiety and bring you into the present moment.
- **Stimulating movements:** Rhythmic cardio bursts, fast-paced walks, or dance energize the body and lighten the mood for those feeling sluggish.
- **Emotional release movements:** Shaking, free-flow dance, and fascia unwinding promote the release of stored emotions and tension in the body.

By experimenting with these movements, you discover what feels most supportive during different emotional states.

Movement Identity: Becoming Someone Who Moves Because It Feels Good

Creating lasting movement habits is about developing an identity that embraces movement as a natural and enjoyable part of who you are. This mindset shift makes movement feel less like a chore and more like a way to honor and care for yourself.

From Motivation to Identity

Motivation is unpredictable and can fluctuate daily due to your mood, energy levels, or other external circumstances. This unpredictability can make relying solely on motivation to maintain a movement routine challenging during perimenopause, when your hormonal shifts already affect your drive and focus.

Rather than relying solely on motivation, developing a movement identity provides a more stable and enduring foundation. This means shifting your self-perception from "I have to work out" to a more empowering mindset like "I am someone who moves regularly because it nourishes my body and mind." When movement becomes part of your identity, it integrates into your lifestyle naturally, rather than feeling like a chore or obligation.

This deeper connection to who you are supports consistency, especially during times when you don't feel motivated. It encourages you to prioritize movement as an expression of self-care and belonging to a healthier, vibrant version of yourself.

Rewriting Your Movement Story

You might carry old beliefs, such as "I'm not sporty" or "Exercise is too hard for me." Changing these narratives helps you build confidence and openness to new forms of movement. Try reframing your inner dialogue:

- "I'm learning to move in ways that suit my body and life."
- "Movement is a way to connect with and celebrate my strength."
- "I choose movement that feels good and supports my well-being."

Anchoring Movement to Your Values

To keep moving consistently during perimenopause, it helps to connect your exercise to what really matters to you. When your workouts reflect your values, they become motivating and meaningful rather than just another thing on your to-do list.

Start by thinking about what's most important in your life. Maybe it's staying healthy and energetic, having strength and focus to enjoy time with family and friends, keeping your mind clear and your mood balanced, or simply caring for yourself and your body. Whatever it is, letting these priorities guide your movement gives you a strong reason to keep going.

For example:

- If spending quality time with loved ones matters most, see your workouts as a way to stay strong and present for them.

- If mental clarity is a priority, consider gentle exercise or mindful movement as a way to clear your head and relieve stress.

- If self-care is your focus, each intentional movement is an act of kindness and appreciation for your body.

This approach helps you pick types of exercise that feel right for you and keeps you motivated even when energy or interest dips. By making your movement personal and meaningful, it becomes a way to honor yourself and what you care about.

Building this kind of movement habit rooted in enjoyment, kindness, and purpose makes it easier to stick with for the long term.

Joyful Movement Menu: Find Your Pleasure Zones

When you move in a way that feels good, you tap into an experience that brings you joy, connection, and satisfaction. Exploring what kinds of movement you enjoy can change how you think about being active and help you build a routine you look forward to.

Discovering What You Enjoy

Different types of movement bring different kinds of pleasure. Take time to notice what sensations and settings make you feel good. Here are some places to start:

- stretching for gentle release and lengthening

- strength training for feeling strong and capable
- rhythmic movement like dancing or walking to music
- moving in nature to connect with fresh air and scenery
- trying novelty or new activities to spark curiosity
- enjoying solitude or quiet movement to tune inwards

The Five Types of Joy in Movement

Understanding the different kinds of joy can help you find what fits best for you:

- **Flow:** getting lost in fluid, effortless movement
- **Connection:** feeling linked to your body, breath, or others
- **Achievement:** reaching a goal or mastering a skill
- **Play:** having fun and being spontaneous
- **Grounding:** feeling steady, safe, and present

Notice which types of joy resonate most and make movement feel rewarding.

Testing and Tweaking Your Movement

Try new activities at a gentle pace to see what feels right. Keep these tips in mind:

- Start small and listen deeply to your body's responses.
- Be curious rather than judgmental about what you like or dislike.

- Build your personalized "joy list" of favorite movements and experiences.
- When boredom, pain, or stress appear, pivot to something different or gentler.

By focusing on pleasure and variety, you create a movement practice that supports your health and happiness, even on challenging days. Your joy menu is a toolkit you can return to whenever movement feels like a struggle.

Daily Movement Energy Check-In and Plan

Use this worksheet daily for a week to tune into your body's energy and decide how to move using the three-lights system.

Step 1: Morning check-in:

- How is my energy level right now?

  ▢ low ▢ moderate ▢ high

- How do my joints and muscles feel?

  ▢ sore ▢ stiff ▢ comfortable ▢ loose

- What symptoms am I noticing?

  ▢ anxiety ▢ brain fog ▢ headaches ▢ hot flashes ▢ none

- What mood am I in?

  ▢ low ▢ neutral ▢ positive

Step 2: Movement decision:

Based on your check-in, tick your movement plan for today:

▢ **Red light:** rest or gentle recovery (breathwork, stretching, or restorative yoga)

▢ **Yellow light:** light movement (mobility, slow walks, or light strength)

▢ **Green light:** regular or intensified workout (strength training, brisk walk, or cardio)

Step 3: Evening reflection

What movement did I do today?

____

____

____

____

How did it feel physically and emotionally?

____

____

____

____

Did my energy or mood change after moving?

____

____

____

____

What adjustments would I make tomorrow?

____

____

____

____

____

Use this daily practice to build a trusting relationship with your body's signals. Over time, you'll become more confident in choosing movement that truly supports your energy and mood each day.

Identify Your Nervous System Movement Type

This reflection helps you discover which nervous system movement pattern fits you best and ways to support yourself through movement. Answer the following:

When I feel anxious or stressed, I usually…

____

____

____

____

____

When I feel low energy or tired, I usually…

____

____

My energy and motivation tend to…

Am I a burner, fader, or drifter? Which of these sounds most like me?

What grounding movements have helped me feel calmer?

What stimulating movements have boosted my energy?

How could I include emotional release movement in my routine?

Action Plan:

Steps I will take to build a nervous-system-smart movement routine:

Movement types I want to experiment with, or include regularly:

Understanding your nervous system type empowers you to select the movement styles that calm, energize, or balance you best. Use this insight to create routines that nurture both your body and mind.

Creating Your Joyful Movement Menu

Explore which movements bring you joy and plan a movement menu to nourish your body and spirit.

Reflect on these questions:

What movements have I enjoyed in the past?

____

____

____

____

____

____

When have I felt most "in the flow" or joyful moving my body?

____

____

____

____

____

What settings or environments inspire me to move?

____

____

____

How do I like to feel before, during, and after movement?

____

Build your Joyful Movement Menu:

List at least five types or styles of movement that bring you pleasure or curiosity. Examples can include stretching, dancing, hiking, swimming, yoga, walking with music, or gardening.

1.
2.
3.
4.

5.

How will I experiment with at least two new or favorite movement types this week?

How will I notice and honor my pleasure zones in movement?

What will I do if movement feels stressful or boring?

Your joyful movement menu is a personalized toolkit to keep your practice fresh, fun, and fulfilling. Return to it often and let pleasure guide your movement choices for lasting motivation.

Final Thoughts

Movement during perimenopause is a journey of listening, adapting, and kindness toward your body. By embracing flexibility, recovery, nervous system awareness, and joy in movement, you create habits that sustain your strength and vitality over time.

Remember that movement should feel good and support your whole well-being, not add stress or pressure. Trust yourself, be patient, and enjoy the process of becoming someone who moves with ease and confidence.

Chapter 11:

Designing Your Life for This Phase—Energy Management, Career Boundaries, and Purpose

Perimenopause often invites you to take a fresh look at how you live your life: how you spend your energy, what you prioritize, and what brings meaning to your days. As your body and mind shift, your lifestyle may need to shift too, so you can feel supported, balanced, and energized.

This chapter will help you notice your natural energy patterns and plan your day around them. You'll learn how to set boundaries that protect your time and energy, both at work and at home. You'll also see how small habits and smart choices can help you stay productive without wearing yourself out. Finally, we'll explore ways to reconnect with what really matters to you, so you can build a life that feels fulfilling and aligned with this stage of life.

By making intentional choices around your work, relationships, and self-care, you can create a life that supports your energy, resilience, and joy, now and in the years to come.

Aligning Your Demands With Your Energy Patterns

One of the biggest keys during perimenopause is learning to work with your body's energy instead of against it. Your energy naturally rises and falls throughout the day, and can shift further across the month as your hormones fluctuate. When you notice and honor these patterns, you can plan your day in a way that feels easier, reduces fatigue, and helps you get more done without burning out.

Tracking Your Energy Rhythms

Start by paying attention to how your energy changes throughout the day and week. You may notice clear times when you feel focused and alert, and other times when you feel drained or foggy. Keep a simple log or journal for several days, noting:

- When during the day am I most productive or clear-headed?
- Are there specific times when I feel more tired or distracted?
- How does my energy change during different points in my menstrual cycle or across the month?

This awareness helps you make smarter choices about when to tackle certain tasks and when to rest.

Task Matching: Aligning Demands to Energy Levels

Once you know your natural energy patterns, you can align your tasks accordingly:

- **High-energy periods:** Tackle tasks that require focus, creativity, or decision-making. Examples of these types of tasks can include writing reports, leading meetings, or solving tricky problems.

- **Low-energy periods:** Save routine or less demanding tasks for these times. This can include answering emails, organizing your space, or handling simple chores.

- **Energy dips:** Schedule restorative activities like gentle movement, meditation, or leisure to recharge without guilt.

Rigid schedules can feel frustrating when your energy isn't at its peak. Stay flexible and allow buffer time for rest or to shift tasks as needed.

Rest and Recharge as Strategic Choices

Rest is an important part of your productivity toolkit. Treating rest as a strategic choice helps you manage energy more sustainably. Take regular breaks during work, use relaxation techniques, or sneak in a short nap if you can. These pauses recharge your body and mind so you can return to tasks feeling refreshed.

By aligning your daily demands with your unique energy rhythms, you work smarter, not harder, while respecting your body's needs. This approach makes it easier to stay balanced and maintain consistent performance through the ups and downs of perimenopause.

Laura's Story: Reclaiming Energy and Purpose

Laura (47) felt drained. Juggling work, family, and household responsibilities left her exhausted and frustrated. She realized her energy didn't match her schedule: mornings, she felt foggy, yet that was when she tackled her hardest tasks; evenings, she had bursts of focus, but little left for self-care or family.

Laura started tracking her energy and noticing patterns. She shifted high-focus work to match her natural peaks, delegated household chores, and said no to extra commitments that drained her. She also identified her core values, balance, creativity, connection, and aligned small habits with them: a 10-minute morning stretch to honor her body, weekly calls with friends, and focused work sprints when her energy was highest.

Over a few months, these simple adjustments rebuilt her sense of agency. Laura regained stability, felt more present, and noticed her daily energy supporting her purpose. By designing her life around her rhythms and values, she moved from overwhelm to a sustainable, fulfilling routine.

Boundary Setting and Saying No with Clarity

Setting boundaries can feel tough. Many of us hesitate to say "no" because we don't want to disappoint others, spark conflict, or seem selfish. But during perimenopause, protecting your energy and well-being is essential for your health and your happiness.

Identifying Your Limits: Building a Clear Foundation

Before you can set boundaries, you need to know what drains you. Tune in to your body and mind and notice the signals that tell you when you're reaching your limit. Ask yourself:

- What can I not give up without feeling depleted?
- When do I start to feel overwhelmed, resentful, or exhausted?
- What signs does my body or mind send before I hit my breaking point?

Write these down. The clearer you are about your limits, the easier it is to protect them.

Communicating Boundaries Assertively and Kindly

Saying no doesn't have to be harsh or apologetic. A few strategies can make it easier:

- Use "I" statements, for example, "I need time to recharge, so I won't be available after 6 p.m."

- Keep it simple and direct. You don't need to over-explain.
- Practice saying "no." Try role-playing with a friend or in front of a mirror to feel more confident.

Your well-being is reason enough. Remember, you don't owe anyone an elaborate justification.

Setting Boundaries in the Workplace

Work can demand too much. Late emails, endless meetings, and multitasking can zap your energy. Here's how to protect yourself:

- Set clear work hours and communicate them to colleagues.
- Learn to say "no" or negotiate deadlines that feel unrealistic.
- Delegate tasks when you can to lighten your load.
- Manage technology by turning off notifications outside work hours to protect your time.

Advocate for yourself while maintaining professionalism and cooperation.

Establishing Boundaries at Home and in Relationships

Family and caregiving responsibilities can take over if you're not careful. Setting boundaries ensures you can give your best without burning out:

- Have honest conversations about what you can and can't take on.
- Ask for help or delegate tasks to others.
- Set rules around communication, like "no phones at dinner" or "quiet time after 9 p.m."

- Be consistent. Calm, steady enforcement teaches long-term respect.

When Boundaries Get Challenged

Boundaries will be tested, especially at first. You may face pushback, guilt-trips, or even doubt yourself. Keep in mind:

- Saying "no" protects your ability to show up fully where it matters most.
- Stand firm and don't feel pressured to repeatedly justify yourself.
- Notice your feelings. If a boundary breach leaves you drained, reinforce it.
- Self-compassion helps you stay calm and confident under pressure.

Setting and keeping clear boundaries is a powerful way to respect yourself and your energy. It gives you the space to thrive during perimenopause and beyond.

Prioritization and Micro Habits for Performance

During perimenopause, managing work, home, and self-care can feel overwhelming. The key to staying productive without burning out is to focus on what really matters and break it down into doable steps.

Using Prioritization Frameworks

Not every task deserves your energy. Prioritization helps you spend time on what truly moves the needle:

- **Use a simple framework**, like the Eisenhower Matrix (Team Asana, 2025):

- urgent and important
- important but not urgent
- urgent but not important
- neither urgent nor important

Focus on the first two categories and consider delegating or minimizing the rest. This keeps your work aligned with your values and reduces overwhelm.

Breaking Tasks Into Micro Habits

Large projects or daily goals can feel daunting. Micro habits turn them into small, easy steps you can do right away.

- Examples can include stretching for a minute, writing a single sentence, or taking three deep breaths before starting.
- These tiny actions build momentum without adding stress.
- They're easy to slip into your existing routines, helping you stay consistent.

Batching and Time Blocking

Grouping similar tasks together keeps your brain focused and reduces mental fatigue:

- Block out time for related activities, such as emails, meetings, or creative work, and stick to it.
- Align these blocks with your peak energy periods for best results.
- When your schedule is structured, you make fewer daily decisions and free up mental space.

This approach keeps your workflow smooth and respects your energy rhythms.

Prioritizing Self-Care as Non-Negotiable

Self-care is a requirement for staying sharp and energized. Here's how to do it:

- Schedule movement, rest, nourishing meals, and good sleep just like appointments.
- Treat them with equal importance as work tasks.
- When you prioritize self-care, you handle your responsibilities with more ease and reduce the risk of burnout.

By combining smart prioritization, small consistent steps, and regular self-care, you can stay productive and energized while honoring your body's changing needs.

Sustaining Meaning and Motivation Post Reset

Once you've made changes to support your health and energy during perimenopause, the next step is keeping your motivation strong and your efforts meaningful. When what you do daily connects with your deeper values, habits stick more easily, and motivation comes naturally.

Clarifying Core Values

Take a moment to reflect on what matters most to you right now. Your values act like a compass, guiding your choices and helping you stay focused when life gets busy or challenging.

Here's how to get clear:

- Journal on prompts like: "What matters most to me?" or "What do I want to stand for?"

- Make a list of your most important values. Examples can include health, family, independence, joy, self-compassion, creativity, balance, or longevity.

- Rank the ones that resonate most with you today.

- Check how your current habits, like movement or self-care routines, align with these top values.

Use this insight to pick or adapt activities that feel meaningful, not just "should-do" tasks. When your choices align with your values, sticking with them becomes easier and more satisfying.

Celebrating Progress and Small Wins

Even tiny wins deserve recognition. Keeping a gratitude or success journal can help you notice achievements, no matter how small.

- Give yourself credit for completing a workout, taking a mindful break, or making a healthy meal choice.

- These positive moments train your brain to associate effort with reward, making habits easier to maintain.

Reframing Challenges as Growth Opportunities

Setbacks are part of the journey. How you view them can make all the difference:

- Instead of labeling difficulties as failures, treat them as learning experiences.

- Reflect on what you can adjust or improve without judging yourself harshly.

- Practice self-compassion, it strengthens your resilience and keeps you moving forward.

Staying motivated is about connecting with your "why" and honoring your journey with kindness. This mindset helps you build lasting change, rather than relying on quick fixes.

Life Design After Perimenopause: Planning Ahead

Perimenopause is a great time to reflect on the future you want to create. Thinking ahead about your well-being, work, relationships, and personal growth helps you design a life that feels fulfilling and balanced.

Envisioning Your Future Self

Imagining who you want to be after perimenopause can make your goals clearer and guide your daily choices:

- Try visualization exercises to picture your ideal lifestyle, health, and relationships.
- Ask yourself questions like, "What does a fulfilling day look like for me?" or "What qualities do I want to embody?"

This vision becomes your guiding star. When you know the life you want, it's easier to make choices today that support it.

Aligning Career Goals With Well-Being

Your work can have a big impact on your energy and satisfaction. Planning a career that fits your health and values ensures your work nourishes rather than drains you:

- Reflect on how to adapt your current role or explore new opportunities with greater flexibility and fulfillment.
- Consider roles like mentorship, consulting, or projects that align with your passions and skills.

- Think about the legacy you want to leave and how your work contributes to it.

When your career aligns with your values, you protect your energy and maintain purpose over the long term.

Strengthening Community and Social Connections

Strong relationships give emotional support and boost overall well-being. You can:

- Focus on people who uplift and energize you.
- Join groups or causes that reflect your interests and values.
- Nurture social ties to protect your mood and resilience through life's changes.

Building strong connections creates a foundation of support and joy that lasts well beyond perimenopause.

Maintaining Adaptability and Growth

Life continues to change after perimenopause. Staying open and curious keeps you engaged and vibrant:

- Accept change as a natural part of life instead of resisting it.
- Check in with yourself regularly to reassess goals, habits, and priorities.
- Explore new interests and skills that enrich your life and keep things fresh.

By planning thoughtfully and staying flexible, you can design a life that's energizing, meaningful, and full of purpose well into the next chapter.

Energy Rhythm Tracking and Task Alignment

Use this worksheet to observe your energy patterns and plan tasks accordingly over one week.

Complete this log daily:

Date: ______________________________

Time of day: ______________________________

Energy level: ______________________________

Mood: ______________________________

Tasks completed: ______________________________

____

____

____

____

____

____

Which tasks felt easier or harder based on energy?

____

____

____

____

____

____

Once you've completed your log, reflect on these questions:

When am I most focused and productive during the day?

___

___

___

___

Which tasks align best with my energy highs?

___

___

___

___

___

___

How can I adjust my schedule to fit these patterns better?

___

___

___

___

___

___

___

What rest or low-energy activities help me recharge effectively?

____

____

____

____

____

____

Next, complete your action plan:

Three changes I will make to align tasks with my energy:

1. ____

____

____

2. ____

____

____

3. ____

____

____

By tracking your energy and aligning tasks thoughtfully, you create a daily rhythm that respects your body's needs and boosts your productivity. Keep returning to this practice to fine-tune your schedule for lasting balance.

Boundary Setting Self-Assessment and Plan

Explore your current boundaries and create an actionable plan to strengthen them. You can use these questions to reflect:

What are my current limits around work, home, and relationships?

____

____

____

____

When have I felt my boundaries were respected? When were they crossed?

____

____

____

____

____

What physical, emotional, or cognitive signs tell me I need stronger boundaries?

____

____

____

____

____

Next, create your boundary-setting plan:

One boundary I want to strengthen or create:

____

____

____

____

How will I communicate this boundary clearly and kindly?

____

____

____

____

____

What challenges might arise, and how will I handle them?

____

____

____

____

____

____

____

____

Who can support me in maintaining this boundary?

____

____

____

____

____

____

Clarifying and communicating your boundaries is a powerful step toward protecting your well-being. Use this plan as a foundation to build stronger boundaries with confidence and compassion over time.

Future Life Vision and Values Clarification

Define your future vision and connect it to your core values for intentional life design. Take a moment to imagine your life five to 10 years from now. Write down:

What does a typical day look like?

____

____

____

____

____

____

How do you spend your time?

____

____

____

____

What relationships and supports are important?

____

____

____

____

____

How do you feel physically, mentally, and emotionally?

____

____

____

Next, reflect on your values:

List your top five core values that support this future vision, for example, balance, creativity, and connection.

1. ____

   ____

   ____

2. ____

3.

4.

5.

How well do your current habits and lifestyle align with these values?

What shifts can you make to better embody your values?

Three intentional changes to move toward your vision:

1. ____

____

____

2. ____

____

____

3. ____

____

____

Your future vision and core values serve as a compass guiding your life choices. Revisit this worksheet whenever you need clarity and inspiration to stay aligned with your true path.

Final Thoughts

Designing your life during and beyond perimenopause is an empowering journey of self-awareness, intention, and compassion. By understanding your energy patterns, setting clear boundaries, prioritizing what truly matters, and connecting deeply with your values and purpose, you create a lifestyle that nurtures your well-being and joy.

Remember, this is your time to design a life that honors who you are and who you are becoming.

Chapter 12:

Your Reset Blueprint—Integrating the Six Pillars, Relapse Prevention, and a Long-Term Vision

You've done something remarkable by getting here. Most women move through perimenopause feeling confused, alone, or overwhelmed. But you showed up for your body, your mind, and your future.

Now it's time to bring everything together into a single, clear plan that supports your long-term health and well-being. Your reset blueprint is built around the six lifestyle pillars we've covered: eating, movement, stress management, sleep, emotions, and addressing imbalances. By combining these elements into a realistic, sustainable approach, you'll feel equipped to handle whatever changes come your way with confidence and resilience.

This chapter will guide you as you create a plan that actually fits your life, helping you manage setbacks with kindness so that occasional slips don't feel like failures. You'll discover ways to track your progress, keep yourself motivated over time, and start shaping long-term goals and a vision for life beyond perimenopause that's thriving, joyful, and balanced.

Your reset blueprint is about taking meaningful steps that honor your body, mind, and spirit every day.

Building a Personalized Reset Plan

Your reset plan is your roadmap for bringing all six lifestyle pillars together in a way that feels doable and meaningful. It helps you stay balanced, build momentum, and adapt as your needs change.

Clarify Your Core Lifestyle Pillars

Start by reflecting on how each pillar currently shows up in your daily life, without judgment:

- How well are you nourishing yourself with whole, balanced foods?
- What does your typical movement or exercise routine look like?
- How do you manage stress and emotional ups and downs?
- What are your sleep habits like in terms of quantity, quality, and routine?
- How well do you handle your emotions and relationships?
- Which imbalances in your life could you address?

Notice which pillars already feel strong and which might need more attention. Remember, these pillars are interconnected: improving sleep can boost mood, managing stress can support digestion, and so on.

Select Achievable Habits

Pick habits that feel doable and bring quick wins or joy:

- Drink an extra glass of water each day.

- Take a short walk after lunch.
- Practice five minutes of deep breathing in the morning.

Start where you feel most motivated or see the biggest need. You don't need to tackle all six pillars at once. Adjust your habits as your body's needs and schedule change.

Link new habits to things you already do. Stretch after brushing your teeth or pause for gratitude before bed. These small connections make it easier to stick with new routines.

Align Habits With Your Values and Priorities

Habits are easier to maintain when they connect to what matters most to you:

- Reflect on your core values. They can include health, family, creativity, independence, or balance. How do your lifestyle choices support them?
- Ask yourself: "Does this habit align with my bigger life goals and who I want to be?"

When your habits resonate with your values, they feel less like chores and more like acts of self-care and self-expression.

Create a Written Plan With Clear Steps

Writing your plan makes your intentions concrete and actionable:

- Outline specific goals for each pillar, along with the habits you want to build. For example, "Move daily with 10 minutes of gentle mobility" or "Practice five-minute breathing exercises three times per week."
- Schedule when and how you'll do each habit, prioritizing consistency but allowing for flexibility.

- Use a planner, app, or journal to include reminders for each pillar and track progress.

- Build in space for reflection and adjustments. Weekly mini-reviews help you notice what's working and what needs tweaking. Ask yourself: Which habits feel natural? Where am I struggling? What can I shift next week?

- Keep your plan visible—on your fridge, desk, or phone—so it's a constant source of motivation and focus.

By creating a personalized, flexible reset plan aligned with your values, you set yourself up for lasting change that supports your body, mind, and life beyond perimenopause.

Maya's Reset in Action

Maya (50) was tired of feeling constantly drained. She took the time to create her reset blueprint, starting with tiny, realistic habits: a five-minute morning stretch, drinking an extra glass of water, and a nightly two-minute gratitude reflection. She aligned these habits with her values of health, connection, and balance.

At first, the changes felt almost invisible, but over a few weeks, Maya noticed a shift. She had more energy during the day, slept better, and felt calmer when unexpected challenges arose. The small habits gave her momentum to tackle slightly bigger changes, like scheduling a weekly walk with a friend and carving out quiet time for reading.

By keeping her plan flexible and celebrating each win, Maya gradually reclaimed her energy, focus, and sense of purpose. What started as a few simple actions became a sustainable lifestyle she could rely on, proving that meaningful change doesn't require a drastic overhaul, just consistent, intentional steps.

Relapse Prevention and Graceful Course Correction

Even with the best plans, life happens. Setbacks are normal, and relapse prevention isn't about never slipping up but rather about handling those moments with kindness and getting back on track without guilt.

Normalize Setbacks as Part of Change

Understand that lapses are a natural part of any lifestyle change. They don't erase your progress. Try these approaches:

- Expect challenges and see setbacks as opportunities to learn what triggers your habits.
- Reframe slips as data, not judgment. Ask yourself: What was happening around me? How was I feeling physically and mentally?
- Avoid harsh self-criticism. Treat yourself as you would a friend.
- Remember that missing a movement session or occasionally eating something less healthy doesn't undo the overall progress you've made.

This mindset creates space for forgiveness, resilience, and the ability to keep moving forward.

Identify Early Warning Signs

Awareness helps you prevent a small slip from becoming a bigger setback.

- Notice patterns or cues that usually come before you stray from your routines.
- Track triggers like fatigue, stress, overwhelm, negative self-talk, or environmental distractions.

- Plan simple responses to interrupt these patterns early.

Knowing your personal warning signs gives you a chance to course-correct before habits unravel.

Build a Supportive Environment

Your surroundings can have a big impact on how you stick to your healthy choices. Consider things like:

- Organize your kitchen, workspace, and living areas to reduce temptations and friction.
- Recruit accountability partners, such as a friend, coach, or support group, to keep you motivated.
- Celebrate small wins and milestones. Positive reinforcement strengthens your habits and mindset.

A supportive environment helps your reset plan stick and makes staying on track feel more natural.

Practice Problem-Solving

Life changes, and so does your body. Flexibility is key when you're problem-solving. Consider things like:

- Adapt your strategies rather than abandoning your efforts. Try new forms of movement, stress-reduction techniques, or modified eating habits if needed.
- Accept that progress isn't a straight line. Ups and downs are normal. Persistence matters more than perfection.
- Stay curious and kind with yourself. Use setbacks to deepen self-awareness and refine your plan.

By embracing relapse prevention and graceful course correction, you maintain momentum without losing self-trust. It's about moving forward with compassion, resilience, and confidence, even when things don't go perfectly.

Trackers and Manifestos for Ongoing Monitoring

Staying aware of your progress and keeping your motivation strong are key to sustaining your reset journey. Using trackers for habits, emotions, and outcomes, along with a personal manifesto, helps you stay connected to your goals and values over time.

Use Comprehensive Habit Trackers

Tracking your habits gives you insight into what supports or hinders your well-being.

- Keep simple logs for each lifestyle pillar: eating, movement, sleep, stress, emotional state, and any imbalances.
- Regular tracking helps you spot trends, celebrate progress, and see where you might need adjustments.
- Include space for notes on successes, challenges, and reflections about what's working for you.
- Trackers can be anything that suits you. This can include charts, apps, journals, or planners.

Incorporate Emotional and Cognitive Check-Ins

Your habits and your mind are connected. Regular check-ins help you notice patterns and refine your approach.

- Use journaling prompts daily or weekly to track mood, focus, and mental clarity.

- Reflect on how your emotions and mindset influence your behaviors.

- Include prompts for gratitude or personal growth to build positivity and resilience.

These reflections strengthen your self-awareness and help you adjust strategies as needed.

Craft a Personal Reset Manifesto

A manifesto is a written statement of your intentions, values, and commitment to yourself.

- Write a declaration that embodies your dedication to well-being, self-kindness, and resilience.

- Include affirmations that reinforce self-trust, empowerment, and compassion.

- Turn to your manifesto when motivation dips or obstacles arise.

- Revisit and revise it regularly to reflect your growth and evolving journey.

Schedule Regular Review Sessions

Set aside time monthly or quarterly to evaluate what's working, what needs tweaking, and how your goals might shift. Update your trackers and your reset blueprint to keep them relevant and motivating.

Using habit trackers, emotional check-ins, and a personal manifesto keeps your reset plan alive and aligned with your evolving body, mind, and purpose. It helps you lead yourself with clarity, intention, and confidence.

Setting and Revisiting Goals for Menopause and Beyond

Building your reset blueprint is just the beginning. To sustain your well-being through menopause and the years that follow, it helps to take a long-term view. Clear goals give you motivation and direction, even when life gets busy or unpredictable.

Develop Long-Term Health and Lifestyle Objectives

Start by thinking about what thriving looks like for you:

- Define broad goals for key areas of life, like maintaining energy, mental sharpness, emotional balance, strong relationships, and self-compassion.
- Structure your goals with the SMART framework:
    - **Specific:** Clearly state what you want, such as improving sleep or staying socially connected.
    - **Measurable:** Decide how you'll track progress, like keeping a sleep journal or logging social activities.
    - **Achievable:** Choose realistic goals that fit your lifestyle.
    - **Relevant:** Make sure your goals align with your values and bigger life vision.
    - **Time-bound:** Set flexible milestones that guide you without adding pressure.

Let your goals evolve as your needs, priorities, and lifestyle change.

Integrate Medical, Psychological and Nutritional Reviews Into Goal Setting

Your health and lifestyle goals work best when paired with regular professional guidance:

- Use check-ups to update treatment plans, screen for changes, and explore symptom management options.

- Stay informed about hormonal therapies, supplements, or lifestyle strategies that could support your well-being.

- Partner with nutritionists or dietitians to refine eating patterns that support hormone and energy balance.

- Come prepared to appointments with questions and goals to make your care align with your reset blueprint.

Combining health monitoring with lifestyle habits strengthens your overall resilience and vitality.

Envision Life Beyond Perimenopause

Life after perimenopause is a chance for growth and renewal. Visualizing the future you want helps guide your daily choices:

- Imagine feeling energized, mentally clear, emotionally balanced, and connected to supportive people.

- Picture how you want to contribute through family, friendships, work, creativity, or community.

- Stay open to the unexpected, seeing changes as opportunities for learning and reinvention.

Use this vision to inspire meaningful goals and decisions that help you reach your fullest potential.

Revisiting your goals with intention and self-compassion turns your reset plan into a lifelong guide for thriving. It empowers you to move through menopause with balance, purpose, and confidence.

Embracing a Long-Term Vision of Thriving

Perimenopause and menopause aren't just about change. They're a chance to grow, discover yourself anew, and create a life that feels energizing and meaningful. By shifting from merely surviving to actively thriving, you open the door to greater self-care, confidence, and control over your health and happiness.

Shift from Survival to Thriving Mindset

Instead of seeing this phase as a time of loss, reframe it as an opportunity:

- Use changes in your body as signals guiding you toward balance and new wisdom.
- Treat challenges as moments to deepen self-awareness and strengthen self-care.
- Celebrate your resilience and capacity to adapt, rather than focusing only on difficulties.

This mindset helps you feel empowered, positive, and capable.

Create Agency Through Knowledge and Compassion

Empower yourself by blending evidence-based understanding with kindness toward yourself:

- Learn how perimenopause affects your body and how lifestyle choices can support your health.
- Replace guilt or self-criticism with curiosity and acceptance when setbacks happen.
- Trust your ability to make decisions that meet your evolving needs.

This combination of knowledge and compassion strengthens your confidence and sense of self-leadership.

Envision a Future Aligned With Your Values

Think about the life you want to lead, guided by what matters most to you:

- Reflect on the legacy, relationships, and purpose you want to nurture.
- Let this vision guide your daily habits and important choices.
- Treat your reset blueprint as a living guide that evolves alongside you.

By embracing a long-term vision of thriving, you give yourself permission to live fully, confidently, and joyfully—through perimenopause, menopause, and all the years beyond.

Personalized Reset Plan Builder

Building a personalized reset plan helps you bring together all the lifestyle changes you've made into one clear, manageable roadmap. This worksheet guides you in assessing your current habits, selecting achievable actions, and aligning your plan with your values to create sustainable, meaningful change.

Step 1: Assess your six lifestyle pillars:

Rate each pillar on a scale of 1–5 based on how well you currently support it in your life (1 = needs lots of attention, 5 = strong and consistent):

- Eating habits: _____
- Movement and exercise: _____

- Stress management: _____
- Sleep quality: _____
- Emotional regulation: _____
- Managing imbalances: _____

Step 2: Choose your habits:

For each pillar, list one or two realistic habits you can start or improve that feel doable and bring you benefits:

Eating habits:

____

____

____

____

____

Movement and exercise:

____

____

____

____

____

Stress management:

Sleep quality:

Emotional regulation:

Managing imbalances:

Step 3: Align with your values:

What are your top three values that your reset plan should support?

1. ______________________________

____

____

2. ______________________________

____

____

3. ______________________________

____

____

How do your chosen habits reflect these values?

____

____

____

____

Step 4: Write your reset plan:

Summarize your plan in a few sentences. Include goals, habits, and how you'll incorporate flexibility.

____

____

____

Use this reset plan as your personalized guide. Revisit and adjust it regularly to honor your evolving needs and sustain your progress.

Relapse Prevention and Graceful Course Correction Plan

Setbacks are a natural part of change, but having a thoughtful relapse prevention plan helps you respond with kindness and resilience. This worksheet helps you identify your triggers, recognize warning signs, and prepare gentle strategies to stay on track or recover smoothly.

Step 1: Identify your common triggers for setbacks:

List situations, feelings, or environments that often challenge your habits:

Step 2: Recognize early warning signs:

What subtle signs alert you that a setback might be approaching? Think physically, emotionally, or behaviorally:

Step 3: Prepare your response strategies:

For each trigger or warning sign, note quick actions you can take to prevent or recover from lapses:

____

Step 4: Support systems:

Who or what can you turn to for encouragement or accountability during challenging times?

____

____

____

____

____

____

____

____

Having a compassionate, clear relapse prevention plan empowers you to navigate setbacks with resilience and keep moving forward gently.

Long-Term Vision and Goal Setting

Setting a long-term vision and clear goals helps you stay motivated and purposeful beyond perimenopause. Use this worksheet to imagine your ideal future, create actionable goals, and plan regular check-ins to stay aligned and adaptable.

Step 1: Envision your life beyond perimenopause:

Write a detailed description of your ideal life 5 to 10 years from now, including health, emotions, relationships, and purpose:

____

Step 2: Define your SMART goals:

Based on your vision, craft three to five long-term goals that are Specific, Measurable, Achievable, Relevant, and Time-bound:

1.

2.

3.

4.

5.

Step 3: Schedule regular check-ins:

How often will you review your goals and progress? What questions will you ask yourself to assess alignment and motivation?

Use this vision and goal-setting worksheet to keep your journey purposeful and adaptable, ensuring that you thrive well beyond perimenopause.

Final Thoughts

Designing and sustaining your personalized reset blueprint is a transformative act of self-care and empowerment. By integrating the six pillars, preparing for setbacks with grace, and setting a clear long-term vision, you lay the foundation for resilience and thriving well beyond perimenopause.

Keep revisiting your plan and goals, celebrate your growth, and embrace the evolving path ahead with confidence and compassion. Remember, this journey is about self-discovery and honoring your body's changing needs. Each small choice, whether it's moving your body, nourishing yourself, taking a mindful pause, or saying "no" to protect your energy, adds up to lasting well-being.

Trust in your ability to adapt, learn, and create routines that feel right for you. Lean on your support system when needed, and give yourself credit for showing up, day after day, for your health, joy, and vitality.

With patience, self-compassion, and intentional action, this phase can become a powerful turning point and a time of renewed energy, clarity, and fulfillment that carries you confidently into the next chapter of your life.

End of Week 8 Reset Manifesto and Next Phase Planning

Let's pause, reflect, and honor the progress you've made so far in your perimenopause reset journey. This collection of worksheets is designed to support you in celebrating your achievements, deepening your self-awareness, and thoughtfully planning how to sustain and build upon your well-being moving forward.

Reflect and Celebrate Your Movement Journey

Movement is more than just physical activity. It's a way to connect with your body, honor its rhythms, and find joy. This exercise will help you recognize the progress you've made.

What movement practices or habits have I developed or strengthened during this reset?

____

____

____

____

Which types of movement energize, calm, or ground me most effectively?

____

____

____

____

How has tuning into my body's nervous system and energy patterns changed my relationship with movement?

____

____

____

____

What is one movement goal or habit I want to continue or deepen into the next phase?

____

____

Write a brief movement reflection and a commitment statement to carry forward.

____

____

____

____

____

____

____

____

____

____

Design Your Life for This Phase

Managing your energy and setting boundaries are key to sustaining health and happiness through this phase. Use this check-in to reflect on how well you align your daily demands with your natural rhythms and how effectively you've protected your time and energy. You'll also identify opportunities to strengthen boundaries moving forward.

What energy patterns have I noticed in my daily and weekly rhythms?

____

____

____

____

How well have I aligned my tasks and priorities to fit these natural energy waves?

____

____

____

____

Which boundaries have I set that support my health and happiness? Which ones need strengthening?

____

____

____

____

What is one practical change or boundary I want to create moving forward?

____

____

How do I see my energy and boundaries? What should be my next step?

____

____

____

____

____

____

____

____

____

____

____

Your Personalized Reset Blueprint Review

Your reset blueprint is your comprehensive guide to sustainable well-being. This exercise invites you to review your plan holistically, examining strengths and areas for growth across the lifestyle pillars. It encourages you to ensure your habits align with your values and to refine your plan for ongoing success.

Which pillars of my reset plan (eating, movement, stress, sleep, emotional well-being, imbalance) feel strongest right now?

____

____

____

____

Where do I notice opportunities to nurture or rebalance these pillars?

____

____

____

____

How do my daily habits reflect my core values and priorities?

____

____

____

____

What small, flexible habit or change can I add or adjust to strengthen my blueprint?

____

____

____

____

Reset Manifesto: Affirming Your Values and Intentions

A personal manifesto is a powerful declaration of your values, intentions, and commitment to yourself. This exercise offers space to articulate your guiding principles and aspirations, serving as a source of inspiration and motivation for the ongoing phases of your journey.

What core values guide my health, well-being, and life choices?

____

____

____

____

____

How do I want to treat myself during challenges and successes?

____

____

____

____

____

What intentions do I hold for my ongoing reset journey and life beyond perimenopause?

____

____

____

____

Planning the Next Phase

Moving beyond the reset phase requires clear vision and actionable goals. This exercise encourages you to envision a thriving future, set meaningful long-term goals, and create a plan for regular check-ins to ensure your continued growth and well-being.

What does thriving look like to me beyond perimenopause?

____

____

____

____

____

What long-term health, emotional, or lifestyle goals inspire me now?

____

____

____

____

What strategies or tools from this reset will I continue using or refining?

____

____

____

____

____

How often will I check in with myself to reflect and adjust my plan?

____

____

____

____

____

Movement Pleasure Portfolio

Joy fuels sustainability. This exercise helps you build a personalized menu of pleasurable movement activities that nourish your body and spirit. Identifying and expanding this portfolio keeps your movement practice enjoyable and dynamic.

List five types of movement activities that bring me pleasure or curiosity.

1. ______________________________________
   ____
   ____
2. ______________________________________
   ____
   ____
3. ______________________________________
   ____
   ____

4. ____

____

____

5. ____

____

____

For each, note what feelings or benefits they evoke, for example, joy, calm, or strength.

____

____

____

____

____

____

Which of these have I incorporated regularly? Which could I try more?

____

____

____

____

____

____

How can I mix or rotate these activities to keep movement exciting and nurturing?

Create a plan to add or try one new pleasurable movement each week for the next month.

Boundary Role Play Preparation

Setting boundaries can be challenging but essential. This exercise supports you in preparing clear, compassionate ways to communicate your limits, boosting confidence and helping you navigate conversations with grace.

Identify one boundary I find hard to assert, either at work, at home, or with friends and family.

____

____

____

____

Write down what makes it difficult, for example, guilt or fear of conflict.

____

____

____

____

____

Draft a clear, compassionate "I" statement to communicate that boundary.

____

____

____

____

Imagine possible responses and prepare how I'll stay firm yet kind.

____

____

____

____

____

____

____

____

Practice this role play with a trusted friend or in front of a mirror until you feel more confident.

Habit Stacking Brainstorm

Building new habits is easier when they are anchored in established routines. This exercise guides you to creatively link healthy practices with daily activities, making consistency more achievable and natural.

List daily routines I already do consistently, for example, brushing teeth, making coffee, or checking email.

____

____

____

____

____

Brainstorm small reset habits I want to build, for example, a one-minute stretch, breath awareness, or drinking water.

Match each new habit to a routine where it naturally fits.

Pick three habit stacks to try in the coming week.

1. ______________________________

____

____

2. ______________________________

____

____

3. ______________________________

____

____

Track how these habit stacks feel and adjust as needed.

Emotional Toolkit Inventory

Emotional regulation is a cornerstone of well-being. This exercise helps you identify your current tools for managing emotions, discover new ones to explore, and plan how to integrate these practices regularly for resilience and balance.

List my go-to methods for calming stress or anxiety, for example, breathing exercises or journaling.

____

____

____

____

Note which have been most effective during perimenopause.

Identify any new emotional practices I want to explore or strengthen.

Plan how to regularly integrate these tools into your routine.

Choose two emotional regulation practices to prioritize this month and schedule reminders.

1. ______________________________

____

____

2. ______________________________

____

____

Reflective Journaling: Progress and Gratitude

Gratitude and reflection foster positivity and motivation. In this exercise, you'll celebrate your wins, acknowledge personal growth, and express appreciation for support, reinforcing a mindset of kindness and perseverance.

What are three things I am proud of accomplishing during my reset journey?

____

____

____

____

____

____

____

____

What unexpected benefits or discoveries have I experienced?

Who or what am I grateful for in supporting this process?

How will I celebrate or honor my progress moving forward?

Write a gratitude note to a supportive person (or myself) who has offered encouragement.

____

____

____

____

____

____

____

____

____

____

____

____

____

____

____

____

____

____

Your reset blueprint is a living document that grows with you. Regularly revisiting and refining your plan keeps it relevant and supportive, empowering you to thrive through ongoing change with intention and kindness.

Preparing for What Comes Next: Menopause Mindset

As you prepare to transition from perimenopause into menopause, this appendix is designed to equip you with the confidence, clarity, and practical tools needed for this next important life stage. While perimenopause sets the foundation for improved self-awareness and lifestyle adjustments, menopause brings its own unique changes and challenges, physically, mentally, and emotionally.

Here, you'll find an overview of what to expect during menopause, including key timelines and common symptoms that differentiate this phase from perimenopause. We'll explore how the six lifestyle pillars you've cultivated continue to support you, and discuss ways to adapt them to meet your evolving needs.

You'll also receive guidance on current medical options, including updates on hormone therapy and the importance of ongoing healthcare partnerships tailored to your personal journey. Strategies for maintaining emotional balance, nourishing nutrition, engaging in purposeful movement, and effective stress management in menopause will be highlighted.

Let's prepare you to embrace menopause with the same empowered mindset and intentional care that has brought you this far.

Overview of Menopause: Key Changes, Timelines, and What to Expect Physically, Mentally, and Emotionally

Menopause marks the natural conclusion of your reproductive years and is officially defined as the point when you've gone 12 consecutive months without a menstrual period. This transition typically occurs between the ages of 45 and 55, but can vary widely. Menopause is a gradual process characterized by significant hormonal shifts that impact your body, mind, and emotions.

Menopause generally unfolds over three phases:

- **Perimenopause:** The transitional period leading up to menopause, lasting several years, characterized by fluctuating hormone levels, irregular cycles, and emerging symptoms.

- **Menopause:** The point in time marking the end of menstrual cycles, diagnosed retrospectively after 12 months without a period.

- **Postmenopause:** The years following menopause, when hormone levels stabilize at lower levels, and symptom patterns may shift again.

Understanding this timeline helps set realistic expectations and prepares you for evolving experiences.

Physical Changes

During menopause, the decline in estrogen and progesterone levels can lead to:

- hot flashes and night sweats

- vaginal dryness and changes in sexual function

- changes in metabolism and body composition, including increased abdominal fat

- bone density loss, increasing osteoporosis risk

- sleep disturbances, including difficulty falling or staying asleep

- increased risk of cardiovascular changes

Each woman's experience is unique. Some may have intense symptoms, while others notice gradual or mild shifts.

Mental and Emotional Changes

Cognitive and emotional shifts are common and can include:

- memory lapses or "brain fog"
- mood swings, irritability, or increased anxiety
- feelings of grief, loss, or identity shifts related to aging and changing roles
- greater introspection and opportunities for personal growth

Hormonal changes influence neurotransmitters that regulate mood and cognition, making these shifts understandable and manageable with the right support and strategies.

What to Expect Emotionally and Mentally

Menopause can be emotionally complex. Some women describe it as a time of liberation and renewed self-awareness, while others may find it challenging to navigate changing feelings and perceived loss. Recognizing this spectrum of responses helps normalize your experience and encourages compassionate self-care.

By understanding the key changes and phases of menopause, you're better prepared to face this transition proactively.

The Six Lifestyle Pillars: Continuing Support and Adaptation During Menopause

The six foundational pillars that have guided your perimenopause reset remain essential as you transition into menopause. However, as your body and life evolve, these pillars may require thoughtful adaptation to meet your changing needs effectively:

- **Eating:** Nutrition continues to play a critical role in managing menopausal symptoms and supporting long-term health. You might find that your metabolism slows further, requiring adjustments to calorie intake or food choices. Prioritize nutrient-dense, anti-inflammatory foods rich in calcium, magnesium, and vitamin D to support bone health. Hydration remains key, and mindful eating can help maintain hormonal balance and emotional well-being.

- **Movement:** Regular physical activity remains a cornerstone for maintaining muscle mass, cardiovascular health, and bone density, all of which may be challenged during menopause. You might need to adjust your exercise routine to focus more on strength training, balance, and flexibility, while continuing to incorporate aerobic and enjoyable movement. Listening to your body's signals and allowing adequate recovery becomes increasingly important.

- **Stress management:** The hormonal shifts of menopause can heighten stress sensitivity, making effective stress management strategies vital. Practices like mindfulness, meditation, breathing exercises, and gentle yoga support nervous system regulation. You may need to deepen or diversify your stress-management toolkit, paying close attention to emotional triggers and ensuring regular self-care breaks.

- **Sleep:** Sleep disturbances often intensify during menopause due to night sweats, hormonal fluctuations, and changing circadian rhythms. Prioritizing sleep hygiene becomes more critical than ever. This might include creating a cooler sleep environment, establishing consistent bedtime routines, limiting stimulants, and utilizing relaxation techniques to improve sleep quality and duration.

- **Emotional regulation:** Emotional shifts may persist or intensify during menopause, making emotional self-leadership essential. Reflective practices, journaling, therapy, and supportive relationships nurture emotional resilience. Adapting your emotional regulation strategies to address mood swings, anxiety, or feelings of loss can help maintain stability and foster growth during this phase.

- **Addressing imbalances in life and habits:** Menopause often brings hormonal shifts as well as changes in lifestyle rhythms and daily habits. This pillar emphasizes identifying and correcting imbalances across physical, emotional, social, and behavioral areas to promote overall well-being. It involves creating awareness of habits that may no longer serve you, such as irregular eating, disrupted sleep patterns, or insufficient self-care, and intentionally restoring balance through sustainable routines. Regularly revisiting and refining your reset blueprint allows you to create harmony in your daily life, supporting your adaptability and resilience during menopause and beyond.

By recognizing that these six pillars remain your steadfast allies and adapting them as your body and life change, you create a resilient foundation for thriving through menopause and beyond. The journey is dynamic, and your toolkit evolves with you, supporting vitality, balance, and joy at every stage.

Strategies for Maintaining Emotional Regulation, Nutrition, Movement, and Stress Management During Menopause

Menopause brings unique challenges that can impact your emotional well-being, nutritional needs, physical activity, and stress levels. Here are practical strategies to help you navigate these areas with care, resilience, and empowerment.

Emotional Regulation

- **Practice mindful awareness:** Regular mindfulness meditation, deep breathing, or grounding exercises can enhance emotional self-awareness and reduce reactive responses.

- **Journaling:** Use journaling to process feelings, track mood fluctuations, and celebrate progress. Reflecting on your emotions helps you identify patterns and triggers.

- **Seek support:** Build connections with supportive friends, family, or professional counselors who understand the menopause journey. Group support or therapy can provide helpful perspectives and coping strategies.

- **Prioritize restorative activities:** Engage in practices like gentle yoga, tai chi, or creative hobbies that soothe your nervous system and promote relaxation.

Nutrition

- **Balance macronutrients:** Prioritize a balance of protein, healthy fats, and complex carbohydrates to support stable blood sugar and hormone balance.

- **Focus on bone health:** Include calcium-rich foods (like leafy greens and fortified products), vitamin D, and magnesium. Consider supplementation if recommended by your healthcare provider.

- **Anti-inflammatory foods:** Incorporate foods high in antioxidants, such as berries, nuts, fatty fish, and colorful vegetables, to reduce inflammation linked to menopausal symptoms.

- **Hydration:** Drink adequate water to combat dryness and support overall metabolic function.

- **Mindful Eating:** Tune into hunger and fullness cues to maintain a healthy weight and cultivate a positive relationship with food.

Movement

- **Incorporate strength training:** Aim for two to three sessions per week to preserve muscle mass and bone density, which naturally decline during menopause.

- **Embrace low-impact aerobic activity:** Walking, swimming, or cycling can improve cardiovascular health while being gentle on joints.

- **Add flexibility and balance work:** Stretching and balance exercises reduce injury risk and enhance mobility.

- **Listen to your body:** Adapt workouts to your energy levels and recovery needs, allowing rest and adjusting intensity as required.

- **Prioritize enjoyable activities:** Engage in movement that feels pleasurable and sustainable to support consistency.

Stress Management

- **Establish daily relaxation rituals:** Build in small moments of calm, such as breathing exercises, meditation, or a brief nature walk. Consistency is key.

- **Set boundaries:** Protect your time and energy by saying no when needed and delegating responsibilities.

- **Use cognitive techniques:** Practice reframing negative thoughts and cultivating self-compassion to reduce the impact of stress.

- **Engage in social connection:** Maintaining supportive relationships helps buffer stress and promotes emotional well-being.

- **Monitor and limit triggers:** Identify stressors like excessive caffeine or poor sleep, and adjust habits accordingly.

Integrating these strategies into your daily life during menopause can enhance your emotional stability, nourish your body, maintain physical vitality, and reduce stress. Combined, they support a balanced, empowered transition characterized by resilience and well-being.

The Importance of Self-Compassion, Ongoing Self-Care, and Revisiting Your Reset Blueprint

Navigating menopause is a dynamic journey that calls for patience, kindness, and a commitment to honoring yourself through each shift and change. Central to thriving during this phase is developing self-compassion. Recognize that fluctuations in mood, energy, and symptoms are natural and not a reflection of personal failure. Treat yourself with the same understanding and care you would offer a close friend facing challenges.

Ongoing self-care is a vital practice for maintaining balance and resilience. This means regularly tuning into your needs and responding with nourishing habits. Self-care might look like prioritizing restful sleep, choosing nutrient-rich foods, taking time for gentle movement, or allowing space for emotional expression and support.

Your personalized reset blueprint is a living, evolving guide designed to adapt as your body and life change. Revisiting and refining it regularly ensures that your lifestyle choices remain aligned with your current needs and aspirations. Whether it's adjusting movement intensity, exploring new stress management techniques, or updating nutrition strategies, staying flexible keeps your plan relevant and effective.

Remember, menopause is a continuing process. Ground yourself in compassion, commit to consistent self-care, and allow your reset blueprint to grow with you.

Menopause Symptom Checklist for Tracking and Awareness

Awareness is the first step to effective management. This symptom checklist is designed to help you regularly observe and track common physical, emotional, and cognitive changes during menopause. Keeping a record not only guides your self-care choices but also enhances communication with healthcare providers.

Use this checklist to monitor common menopausal symptoms. Regular tracking helps you notice patterns, communicate effectively with healthcare providers, and tailor your lifestyle strategies.

- ▢ hot flashes or sudden heat sensations
- ▢ night sweats disrupting sleep
- ▢ irregular periods or changes in bleeding patterns
- ▢ vaginal dryness or discomfort
- ▢ changes in libido or sexual function
- ▢ sleep disturbances, including insomnia or restless sleep
- ▢ mood swings, irritability, or increased anxiety
- ▢ memory lapses or difficulty concentrating
- ▢ fatigue or low energy
- ▢ weight changes, especially increased abdominal fat

▢ joint or muscle aches

▢ dry skin or hair changes

▢ urinary urgency or incontinence

▢ headaches or migraines

▢ breast tenderness

Use this checklist as a flexible tool. Check in regularly, note new or shifting symptoms, and celebrate progress. Tracking empowers you to respond thoughtfully and proactively as your menopause journey unfolds.

Adapting Your Reset Framework to Menopause

Your reset blueprint is a dynamic guide that grows with you. This planning worksheet encourages you to revisit and adapt your lifestyle strategies specifically for menopause, ensuring your habits and goals continue to support your health, balance, and vitality during this new phase.

Review Your Current Reset Blueprint

Which pillars remain strong and supportive?

____

____

____

____

____

Where are my greatest challenges during menopause?

Identify Necessary Adaptations

What changes or new habits can support emerging symptoms or shifting priorities?

How might I adjust my nutrition, movement, stress management, sleep, emotional regulation, or hormonal strategies?

Set Specific Goals

Define two to three clear, achievable goals tailored to my menopause experience. Include timelines and ways I will measure progress.

Support and Resources

List people, healthcare providers, community groups, or tools I can engage with for encouragement and guidance.

Self-Care Commitment

What daily or weekly self-care actions will I prioritize to nurture my well-being?

Revisit this plan periodically to reflect on what's working and where I may need adjustments. Your proactive planning cultivates ongoing empowerment and resilience throughout menopause.

Mindset Shifts and Readiness for the Next Phase

Menopause is as much a mental and emotional journey as it is physical. These reflection prompts invite you to explore your mindset, acknowledge your feelings, and foster readiness for the changes ahead with curiosity and self-compassion.

How has my perspective on menopause evolved through my perimenopause journey?

____

____

____

____

____

____

What aspects of this transition am I welcoming with openness?

____

____

____

____

____

____

Where do I feel resistance or fear, and how might I approach these feelings with compassion?

What strengths and skills have I developed that will support me in menopause?

How can I continue to nurture a growth mindset as I face new experiences?

What ongoing practices will help me stay connected to my values and intentions?

How will I celebrate my resilience and progress during this next chapter?

Use these prompts as a regular practice in journaling or conversation to nurture a positive, growth-oriented mindset. Embracing reflection helps you meet menopause with openness and strength.

As you move forward, remember that the six pillars you've created continue to offer powerful support, even as your needs evolve. Tracking your symptoms, revisiting your reset blueprint, and embracing strategies tailored to this phase empower you to navigate menopause with confidence and resilience.

You're now part of a growing community of women rewriting the narrative around midlife and menopause, embracing it as a time of renewal and strength. May you continue to embody your reset with confidence and joy, advocate for your health, and inspire others through your lived example.

Conclusion

You've reached the end of this book, yet in truth, you are standing at the threshold of a new chapter in your life. Perimenopause can feel confusing, even disruptive, but by learning, exploring, and choosing a path of empowerment, you've already taken a remarkable step.

This phase of life is more than just a collection of symptoms to endure. It's an invitation to reset habits, reconnect with your body, and build steadier foundations for the years ahead. The six lifestyle pillars are your tools: small, flexible steps that guide your system back into balance.

Celebrate this commitment. You've joined a growing community of women redefining midlife by choosing strength, clarity, and grace over confusion and silence. Keep your reset plan close, let your trackers and reflections evolve, and seek support from communities and health professionals who honor your voice.

Share your journey with others to help them use this phase of life as a reset. Every honest conversation breaks stigma, helping another woman feel seen and supported. This is how we transform midlife: from something to endure into something to embrace.

Carry these tools with care. Move with intention, honor your needs, and lead your well-being with compassion. Let this chapter be your ritual of renewal: a daily act of listening, adjusting, and celebrating yourself.

Rise with steadiness. Thrive with intention. Shine with the vitality of your evolving self. The journey continues, and you are ready.

References and Further Reading

The sources below include both works cited directly in this book and additional research that informed its development. They are offered as a resource for readers who wish to explore these topics more deeply.

Akers, A. (2023, August 3). *Preventing burnout: 7 strategies and when to seek help*. Medical News Today. https://www.medicalnewstoday.com/articles/preventing-burnout

Arnison, S. (2025, September 28). *Six pillars of lifestyle medicine*. Ascot Menopause. https://ascotmenopause.com/six-pillars-of-lifestyle-medicine

Baker, J. H., Eisenlohr-Moul, T., Wu, Y.-K., Schiller, C. E., Bulik, C. M., & Girdler, S. S. (2019). Ovarian hormones influence eating disorder symptom variability during the menopause transition: A pilot study. *Eating Behaviors*, *35*, 101337. https://doi.org/10.1016/j.eatbeh.2019.101337

Bendis, P. C., Zimmerman, S., Onisiforou, A., Zanos, P., & Georgiou, P. (2024). The impact of estradiol on serotonin, glutamate, and dopamine systems. *Frontiers in Neuroscience*, *18*. https://doi.org/10.3389/fnins.2024.1348551

Brown, C. M. (2025, April 25). *Menopause cravings: Hormones and appetite*. Winona. https://bywinona.com/journal/menopause-cravings-the-connection-between-hormones-and-appetite?srsltid=AfmBOop7n6qXOH9OCMNt0dM_Bq5d093QTfX3NOGZ5QFnmgYkHShvqpT6

Brown, L. (2017, June 29). *Self-compassion may help women cope with menopausal symptoms.* The University of Melbourne. https://pursuit.unimelb.edu.au/articles/self-compassion-may-help-women-cope-with-menopausal-symptoms

Calcium. (2025, July 11). National Institutes of Health. https://ods.od.nih.gov/factsheets/Calcium-HealthProfessional/

Caraher, E. (n.d.). *The difference between physical hunger and emotional hunger.* Northwell Mather Hospital. https://www.matherhospital.org/weight-loss-matters/the-difference-between-physical-hunger-and-emotional-hunger/

Carefoot, H. (2025, October 30). *6 lifestyle changes improve menopause symptoms, experts say.* Flow Space. https://www.theflowspace.com/reproductive-health/menopause/lifestyle-changes-menopause-symptoms-3008972/

Caring for your skin in menopause. (2023, November 20). American Academy of Dermatology Association. https://www.aad.org/public/everyday-care/skin-care-secrets/anti-aging/skin-care-during-menopause

Cauley, J. A. (2015). Estrogen and bone health in men and women. *Steroids, 99,* 11–15. https://doi.org/10.1016/j.steroids.2014.12.010

Cepni, A. B., Ma, H. Y., Irshad, A. M., Yoe, G. K., & Johnston, C. A. (2024). Addressing shame through self-compassion. *American Journal of Lifestyle Medicine.* https://doi.org/10.1177/15598276241292993

Chong, J., & Collyer, J. (2024, March). Perimenopause: What it is and how to cope with the physical and emotional impact. *The Skill*

Collective. https://theskillcollective.com/blog/perimenopause-signs

Clear, J. (n.d.). *The ultimate habit tracker guide: Why and how to track your habits.* James Clear. https://jamesclear.com/habit-tracker

Coslov, N., Richardson, M. K., & Woods, N. F. (2023). "Not feeling like myself" in perimenopause — what does it mean? Observations from the Women Living Better survey. *Menopause*, 10.1097/GME.0000000000002339. https://doi.org/10.1097/GME.0000000000002339

Cunningham, S. (2025, March 31). *Rest and recovery are critical for an athlete's physiological and psychological well-being.* UCHealth. https://www.uchealth.org/today/rest-and-recovery-for-athletes-physiological-psychological-well-being/

Dias, R. K. N., Penna, E. M., Noronha, Á. S. N., Neto, O. B., Monteiro, E. P., & Coswig, V. S. (2024). Minimal dose resistance training enhances strength without affecting cardiac autonomic modulation in menopausal women: a randomized clinical trial. *Scientific Reports*, *14*(1), 19355. https://doi.org/10.1038/s41598-024-69073-4

Dick, B. (2025, September 11). Rediscovering your "why": Finding purpose and passion in your 40s. *Bonafide.* https://hellobonafide.com/blogs/news/finding-purpose-menopause

Digitale, E. (2024, May 16). *Mental health and menopause: There are connections and solutions.* Stanford Medicine. https://med.stanford.edu/news/insights/2024/05/mental-health-menopause-perimenopause-solutions.html

Dodson, M. (2025, October 1). Perimenopause to menopause: Reclaiming restful sleep. *One Medical.*

https://www.onemedical.com/blog/preventive-care/perimenopause-to-menopause-reclaiming-restful-sleep/

Dutchen, S. (2021). *The mental health aspects of menopause.* Harvard Medicine Magazine. https://magazine.hms.harvard.edu/articles/mental-health-aspects-menopause

Dweck, C. (2017). *Mindset: Changing the way you think to fulfill your potential.* Robinson.

Edwards, K. M., & Mills, P. J. (2008). Effects of estrogen versus estrogen and progesterone on cortisol and interleukin-6. *Maturitas,* *61*(4), 330–333. https://doi.org/10.1016/j.maturitas.2008.09.024

Erbil, N. (2018). Attitudes towards menopause and depression, body image of women during menopause. *Alexandria Journal of Medicine,* *54*(3), 241–246. https://doi.org/10.1016/j.ajme.2017.05.012

Erdélyi, A., Pálfi, E., Tűű, L., Nas, K., Szűcs, Z., Török, M., Jakab, A., & Várbíró, S. (2024). The importance of nutrition in menopause and perimenopause — A review. *Nutrients,* *16*(1), 27. https://doi.org/10.3390/nu16010027

Fenske, S. (2025, September 1). *Circadian rhythm and sleep in perimenopause.* Tara MD. https://www.taramd.com/post/circadian-rhythm-and-sleep-in-perimenopause

Fry, A. (2025, July 29). *Sleep, athletic performance, and recovery.* Sleep Foundation. https://www.sleepfoundation.org/physical-activity/athletic-performance-and-sleep

Gastman, S., & Hanan, M. (2023, May 30). *How menopause can impact your relationship with food.* Dietetically Speaking.

https://dieteticallyspeaking.com/how-menopause-can-impact-your-relationship-with-food/

Hanna, C. (2025, January 21). Guide to boosting body image during menopause. *Versalie.* https://www.versalie.com/blogs/learn/body-image-during-menopause

Harland, N. (n.d.). *Physical vs emotional hunger: understanding the key differences.* Numan. https://www.numan.com/weight-loss/diet/physical-vs-emotional-hunger-key-differences

Harper-Harrison, G., Shanahan, M. M., & Carlson, K. (2024). *Hormone replacement therapy.* National Library of Medicine. https://www.ncbi.nlm.nih.gov/books/NBK493191/

Hassing, S. (2025, September 14). *22 high protein high fiber meals.* The Real Food Dietitians. https://therealfooddietitians.com/high-protein-high-fiber-meals/

Haver, M. C. (2024, April 30). *Your complete guide to finding excellent menopause care.* Oprah Daily. https://www.oprahdaily.com/life/health/a60527187/guide-to-finding-menopause-treatment/

Haufe, A., & Leeners, B. (2023). Sleep disturbances across a woman's lifespan: What is the role of reproductive hormones? *Journal of the Endocrine Society*, *7*(5). https://doi.org/10.1210/jendso/bvad036

Hirschberg, A. L. (2012). Sex hormones, appetite and eating behaviour in women. *Maturitas*, *71*(3), 248–256. https://doi.org/10.1016/j.maturitas.2011.12.016

Isenmann, E., Kaluza, D., Havers, T., Elbeshausen, A., Geisler, S., Hofmann, K., Flenker, U., Diel, P., & Gavanda, S. (2023). Resistance training alters body composition in middle-aged women depending on menopause - A 20-week control trial. *BMC Women's Health*, *23*(1). https://doi.org/10.1186/s12905-023-02671-y

Klynn, B. (2024, November 28). Emotional regulation: Skills, exercises, and Strategies. *BetterUp*. https://www.betterup.com/blog/emotional-regulation-skills

Lang, A. (2024, November 27). *10 natural ways to balance your hormones*. Healthline. https://www.healthline.com/nutrition/balance-hormones

Lewis, H. (2024, November 12). *How to set boundaries at work – with examples*. Halo Psychology. https://halopsychology.com/2024/11/12/how-to-set-boundaries-at-work-with-examples/

Liu, A. (2025, March 18). *Perimenopause and menopause and your mental health: What you need to know*. Lukin Center for Psychotherapy. https://www.lukincenter.com/perimenopause-and-menopause-and-your-mental-health-what-you-need-to-know/

Lovink, R. (2025, November 4). *Understanding perimenopause and gut health*. Canadian Digestive Health Foundation. https://cdhf.ca/en/understanding-perimenopause-and-gut-health/

Lubeck, B. (2025, August 25). *18 herbs and supplements for balanced hormones*. Verywell Health. https://www.verywellhealth.com/can-supplements-help-balance-your-hormones-7965924

Lutich, A. (2024, August 2). Menopause is having a moment: Debunking common myths. *UT Southwestern Medical Center*. https://utswmed.org/medblog/menopause-myths/

MacAvoy, S., & Clasen Marsanico, T. (2025, February). *28 easy high-protein, high-fiber meals for all your health goals.* Good Housekeeping. https://www.goodhousekeeping.com/food-recipes/healthy/g63350024/high-protein-high-fiber-meals/

Marks, J. L. (2025, August 6). *10 tips to manage menopausal fatigue.* Everyday Health. https://www.everydayhealth.com/hs/guide-to-managing-menopause/8-energy-boosters-for-menopause-fatigue/

Matza, S. (2025, April 14). Why comfort food cravings intensify during perimenopause. *Patients like Me.* https://www.patientslikeme.com/blog/perimenopause-hunger-food-cravings

McGarvie, S. (2025, January 9). *Emotional regulation: 5 evidence-based regulation techniques.* Positive Psychology. https://positivepsychology.com/emotion-regulation/

McIntyre, R. (2024, April 17). How to practise self-compassion during menopause. *VHi.* https://www1.vhi.ie/blog/articles/how-to-practise-self-compassion-during-menopause

Melatonin. (2025, April 28). Cleveland Clinic. https://my.clevelandclinic.org/health/articles/23411-melatonin

Melemis, S. M. (2015). Relapse prevention and the five rules of recovery. *The Yale Journal of Biology and Medicine*, *88*(3), 325. https://pmc.ncbi.nlm.nih.gov/articles/PMC4553654/

Menefee, D. S., Ledoux, T., & Johnston, C. A. (2022). The importance of emotional regulation in mental health. *American Journal of Lifestyle Medicine*, *16*(1), 28–31. https://doi.org/10.1177/15598276211049771

Metcalf, C. A., Duffy, K. A., Page, C. E., & Novick, A. M. (2023). Cognitive problems in perimenopause: A review of recent evidence. *Current Psychiatry Reports*, *25*(10), 501–511. https://doi.org/10.1007/s11920-023-01447-3

Migala, J. (2024, December 6). *Menopause diet plan: What to eat during menopause.* Midi. https://www.joinmidi.com/post/menopause-diet-plan

Musial, N., Ali, Z., Grbevski, J., Veerakumar, A., & Sharma, P. (2021). Perimenopause and first-onset mood disorders: A closer look. *Psychiatry Online*, *19*(3), 330–337. https://doi.org/10.1176/appi.focus.20200041

Nappi, R. E. (2025). Lifestyle medicine: a must-have in the menopause toolkit. *Climacteric*, *28*(5), 475–477. https://doi.org/10.1080/13697137.2025.2549207

Newson, L. (2024, December 30). *How to set goals to boost your health and happiness.* Dr Louise Newson. https://www.drlouisenewson.co.uk/knowledge/how-to-set-goals-to-boost-your-health-and-happiness

Nichols, H. (2025, April 22). *Estrogen: Functions, uses, and imbalances.* Medical News Today. https://www.medicalnewstoday.com/articles/277177

Park, K. M. (2024, August 13). *Sleep disturbance in perimenopausal women.* Chronobiology in Medicine. https://www.chronobiologyinmedicine.org/m/journal/view.php?number=182

Patil, R. C., & Unverferth, K. (2023, October 24). *Treating the mental health side of menopause.* UCLA Health. https://www.uclahealth.org/news/article/treating-mental-health-side-menopause

Perimenopause. (2024, August 8). Cleveland Clinic. https://my.clevelandclinic.org/health/diseases/21608-perimenopause

Perimenopause. (2025, August 14). Mayo Clinic. https://www.mayoclinic.org/diseases-conditions/perimenopause/symptoms-causes/syc-20354666

Peters, B., Santoro, N., Kaplan, R., & Qi, Q. (2022). Spotlight on the gut microbiome in menopause: Current insights. *International Journal of Women's Health, Volume 14*(14), 1059–1072. https://doi.org/10.2147/ijwh.s340491

The perimenopause timeline: how long it lasts and what happens. (2025, February 28). Evernow. https://www.evernow.com/learn/the-perimenopause-timeline?srsltid=AfmBOoogFpV8PXNNa0enYt6a7VR38UJJKrnAMVNkmZSs01-UwF4sfy3n

Perry, E. (2023, December 19). The 11 best habit tracker apps to build new behaviors. *BetterUp.* https://www.betterup.com/blog/best-habit-tracker-apps

Pinelli, K. (2025, October 28). *How perimenopause impacts your sense of self—and how to reclaim it.* Rust Wellness Group. https://www.rustwellnessgroup.com/how-perimenopause-impacts-your-sense-of-self-and-how-to-reclaim-it

Progesterone changes in perimenopause. (2024, April 1). Tara MD. https://www.taramd.com/post/progesterone-changes-in-perimenopause

Santoro, N., Epperson, C. N., & Mathews, S. B. (2015). Menopausal symptoms and their management. *Endocrinology and Metabolism Clinics of North America, 44*(3), 497–515. https://doi.org/10.1016/j.ecl.2015.05.001

Scaccia, A. (2022, July 3). *Serotonin: Functions, side effects, and more.* Healthline. https://www.healthline.com/health/mental-health/serotonin

Sexual health. (n.d.). The Menopause Society. https://menopause.org/patient-education/menopause-topics/sexual-health

Silver, N. (2023, April). *Mood changes during perimenopause are real. Here's what to know.* Every Stage Health. https://www.acog.org/womens-health/experts-and-stories/the-latest/mood-changes-during-perimenopause-are-real-heres-what-to-know

Smith, C. (2024, December 3). *Perimenopause tiredness: Managing menopause fatigue.* The Women's Clinic. https://www.thewomensclinic.co.uk/perimenopause-tiredness-managing-menopause-fatigue/

Smith, M., Robinson, L., & Segal, J. (2025, January 16). *Emotional eating and how to stop it.* HelpGuide.org. https://www.helpguide.org/wellness/weight-loss/emotional-eating

Somers, D. L. (2025, June 16). Menopause and sleep: How to get a better night's rest. *Temple Health.* https://www.templehealth.org/about/blog/menopause-and-sleep

Stafford, E. (2025, May 1). *The power of prioritization: How to work smarter, avoid burnout and drive real impact.* Forbes. https://www.forbes.com/councils/forbesbusinesscouncil/2025/05/01/the-power-of-prioritization-how-to-work-smarter-avoid-burnout-and-drive-real-impact/

Stasnopolis, A. (2025, July 14). Hormone-balancing diet: Top foods that help balance hormones. *Scrubbing In.* https://www.bswhealth.com/blog/hormone-balancing-diet

Stewart, M. (2023, May 1). *How to handle menopause brain fog.* National Council on Aging. https://www.ncoa.org/article/how-to-handle-menopause-brain-fog/

Stone, E. (n.d.). Perimenopause and fatigue: Tips for boosting your energy levels. *Virginia Physicians for Women.* https://vpfw.com/blog/perimenopause-and-fatigue-tips-for-boosting-your-energy-levels/

Sutton, J. (2021, July 24). *How to boost self-esteem: 12 simple exercises and CBT tools.* Positive Psychology. https://positivepsychology.com/self-esteem-boost-exercises/

Sutton, J. (2022, February 1). *How to change behavior and habits: 15 therapy techniques.* Positive Psychology. https://positivepsychology.com/behavior-change-techniques/

Team Asana. (2025, January 29). *The Eisenhower matrix: How to prioritize your to-do list.* Asana. https://asana.com/resources/eisenhower-matrix

Watson, S., & Cherney, K. (2025, May 1). *The effects of sleep deprivation on your body.* Healthline. https://www.healthline.com/health/sleep-deprivation/effects-on-body

Way, G. (2025, June 27). *Best skin care for menopausal skin.* Midi. https://www.joinmidi.com/post/best-skincare-for-menopausal-skin

Welch, A. (2024, July 23). *30-second breath work exercises you can do anywhere.* EverydayHealth.

https://www.everydayhealth.com/integrative-health/breathwork-exercises-you-can-do-anywhere/

West, E. (2025, March 11). Nutritional tips for perimenopausal and menopausal women. *Eileen West MD and Associates.* https://www.eileenwestmd.com/blog/perimenopause-and-menopause-nutrition-tips/

Woods, N. F., Mitchell, E. S., & Smith-DiJulio, K. (2009). Cortisol levels during the menopausal transition and early postmenopause. *Menopause, 16*(4), 708–718. https://doi.org/10.1097/gme.0b013e318198d6b2

Yazdkhasti, M., Simbar, M., & Abdi, F. (2015). Empowerment and coping strategies in menopause women: A review. *Iranian Red Crescent Medical Journal, 17*(3). https://doi.org/10.5812/ircmj.18944

Zhang, T. (n.d.). *Navigating perimenopause: 5 tips from a women's health provider.* Johns Hopkins Medicine. Retrieved November 16, 2025, from https://www.hopkinsmedicine.org/health/wellness-and-prevention/navigating-perimenopause-5-tips-from-a-womens-health-provider.

www.ingramcontent.com/pod-product-compliance
Lightning Source LLC
LaVergne TN
LVHW100513110826
845146LV00002B/619

* 9 7 9 8 9 9 6 3 4 9 1 0 4 *